I Can't Believe It's Yoga!

If you are one of the millions of Americans who have heard about the wonderful benefits of Yoga, but have never tried it, this book is for you.

It offers a simple and effective way to:

- Improve your flexibility
- Tone and strengthen your muscles
- Relax your body

After just a few short weeks, you'll feel so great that you too won't believe it's Yoga.

I Can't Believe It's Yoga!

Lisa Trivell

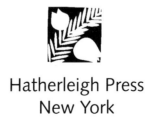

Hatherleigh Press
New York

A Getfitnow.com Book

I Can't Believe It's Yoga
A Getfitnow.com Book

Hatherleigh Press/Get fitnow.com Books
An Affiliate of W.W. Norton & Company, Inc
5 - 22 46th Avenue
Long Island City, NY 11101
1-800-528-2550

Visit our website: www.getfitnow.com

Disclaimer:

Before beginning any strenuous exercise program consult your physician. The
author and publisher of this book and workout disclaim any liability, personal or
professional, resulting from the misapplication of any of the training procedures
described in this publication.

All Getfitnow.com titles are available for bulk purchase, special
promotions, and premiums. For more information, please contact the manager
of our Special Sales Department at 1-800-528-2550.

Library of Congress Cataloging-in-Publication Data
Trivell, Lisa, 1956-
    I can't believe it's yoga! / Lisa Trivell.
        p.   cm.
    ISBN 1-57826-26-032-9 (alk. paper)
    1. Yoga--Therapeutic use.   2. Yoga--Health aspects.
RM727.Y64T75   1999
613.7'046--dc21   99-33649
                                                                        CIP

Cover design by Lisa Fyfe
Text design and composition by dcdesigns

Photographed by Peter Field Peck
with Canon® cameras and lenses on Fuji® slide film
Printed in Canada on acid-free paper
10 9 8 7 6 5 4

I dedicate this book to the love and support of my husband Jim, and my children Amanda and Dylan.

Acknowledgements

I would like to give a special thanks to Tracy Tumminello, for her patience, encouragement, and editing talent.

My publisher Andrew Flach, for his vision that made this project come to life.

Peter Field Peck, for his magnificent photography.

I am grateful to my first Yoga teachers, Eleanor Goff, Elaine Summers, Emily Conrad, and Sidi Hessel.

I would like to thank my most recent teachers and colleagues, Patia Cunningham, Marni Task, Tesh, Jessica Bellofatto, and Kevin Gardiner.

I am appreciative of all the students and clients in my massage and Yoga practice.

CONTENTS

PART I: INTRODUCTION

I am not sure if this Yoga stuff is for me.

Everyone can benefit from the numerous advantages of Yoga. You'll see.

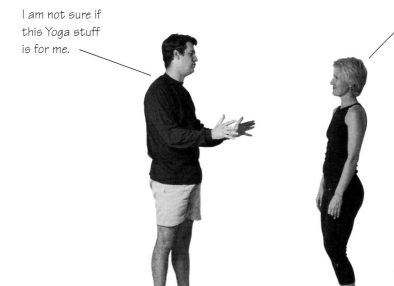

This program is perfect for beginners.

I have been interested in trying Yoga for quite some time.

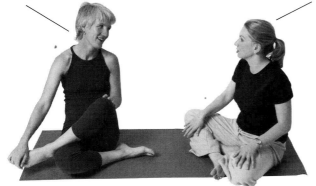

Yoga has gained renewed respect and interest in the last few years for the way it integrates concentration, stretching, strength training, and balance. More and more people have heard of the benefits of Yoga and are curious and willing to try it.

I Can't Believe It's Yoga is a simple program that anyone can do, regardless of their experience or fitness level. Everyone *can* and *should* benefit from the numerous advantages of Yoga. I guarantee that after doing Yoga for only a couple of weeks, you will feel so great both mentally and physically, you will want to continue to practice Yoga regularly.

Yoga is different from other forms of fitness because it is performed with an inward focus. The Yoga taught in this book is performed at a slow pace, emphasizing quality of movement and correct positioning. These activities are process-oriented, achieved by focusing on the movements. It is important to pay attention to your individual needs in order to benefit the most from your Yoga workout.

Often times, many people still feel muscle soreness after their regular workouts. Doing ten minutes of Yoga after going to the gym can help stretch and relax tired muscles.

The more you do Yoga, the easier it becomes and the more you get from it. I have many students that never practiced Yoga before they came to my class. These students do Yoga alongside more advanced students and, since the focus is inward rather than competitive, they learn from one another.

We can all benefit from adding Yoga to our fitness routines:

- *For a mother running around all day who may feel tired, out of shape, and stressed, Yoga is the perfect workout. She can take ten minutes out three times a week to lay on her mat, ignore the telephone, and do Yoga. Yoga will calm her nerves, give her energy, and tone her muscles.*

- *Yoga can also help a busy executive relax at the end of the day. He will find that if he takes time out to do Yoga's guided relax ation, he will unwind, de-stress, and sleep more soundly.*

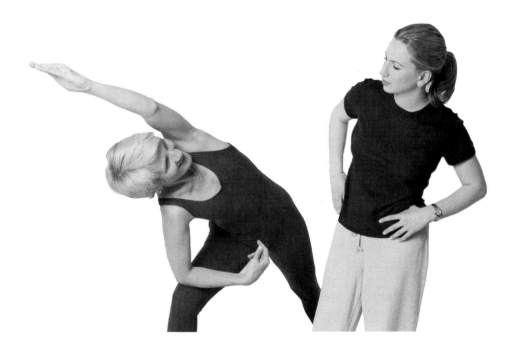

• *Yoga can even help the college student hunched over a desk, staring at a computer screen while working on a paper. Taking a ten-minute break to do Yoga can help revitalize dwindling energy, relax strained eyes, and release back tension.*

If you have been skeptical about Yoga in the past, fear not. In these pages you will discover a simple and effective way to make Yoga a vital part of a healthier lifestyle.

And please, if you have any questions regarding this book, please visit the getfitnow.com website and post them in the *I Can't Believe It's Yoga* Discussion Forum. I'll be happy to reply! Good luck.

–Lisa Trivell

PART II: WHAT IS YOGA?

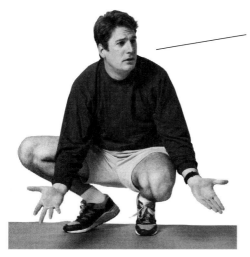

Yoga? What can it do for me?

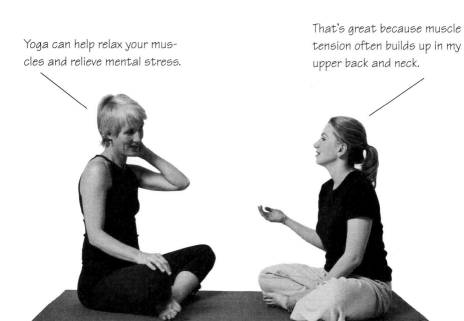

Yoga can help relax your muscles and relieve mental stress.

That's great because muscle tension often builds up in my upper back and neck.

A Brief History of Yoga

Yoga, an ancient art of movements, originated from the practices of spiritual seekers in India. For over six thousand years, Yoga has been used to strengthen and energize for long hours of meditation. Although we do not all intend to live on an ashram and meditate, we can take advantage of Yoga's benefits for different purposes. We can use the techniques of Yoga to help center, strengthen, and energize ourselves.

This book is based on the Yoga teachings of Hatha. Although Hatha is not a religious practice, there are underlying concepts designed to help people develop balance and harmony with the world around them.

The word "Yoga" means union. Hatha Yoga helps define the importance of the push and pull in the universe, such as the Sun and the Moon. This is an example of a union of equal opposites. This also helps us understand the union between the individual self and the universe. Smooth deep breaths are synchronized with the movements, which helps purify and realign the body to cultivate a feeling of inner peace.

How Can It Help

In our daily lives, muscles are often habitually contracted due to sitting long hours at a desk, driving cars, and carrying bags unevenly. Yoga teaches you how to elongate your muscles. Not only will you learn to use the larger muscles of your body, but you will also begin to focus on smaller muscles, tendons, and joints. You often reawaken muscles you were not even aware you had while doing Yoga. The goals of Yoga are to achieve suppleness, agility, revitalized body sensitivity, increased muscle shape and tone, and a state of released mental stress.

After doing Yoga regularly three times a week for 10 minutes, and one time during the weekend for 30 minutes, you will sense a lightness in the way your body feels, looks, and moves.

These dynamic exercises will help you develop power and control.

Yoga will help you strengthen weak muscle groups and learn to activate neglected support muscles, both essential elements in developing good posture.

These dynamic exercises will help you develop power and control. Yoga will help you strengthen weak muscle groups and learn to activate neglected support muscles, both essential elements in developing good posture.

BENEFITS

Benefits Include:
* Relaxes muscle tension.
* Gently speeds your cardiovascular system.
* Great to add to a cross-training program.
* Provides benefits similar to those of a massage.
* Creates time out from busy day.
* It is non-competitive.
* You can practice it all your life.
* You will look and feel younger.
* Improves skin tone and complexion.
* Time and energy efficient.
* Reduces strain on muscles due to overexertion.
* Increases strength and flexibility.
* Increases self-confidence.
* Creates posture awareness.
* Teaches you relaxation techniques that can lower blood pressure.
* Strengthens your immune system.
* Tones your organs.

Different Yoga exercises channel blood flow into specific areas of the body. The increased circulation to an area of the body helps to nourish that area and promote better health. The body is made up of ten systems, each of which benefit from this workout:

1. **Skeletal** – Bones will increase in strength, helping to improve posture.

7

2. **Muscular** – Muscles are stretched and toned. Yoga warms up all the muscles groups, even the ones you don't normally use.

3. **Circulatory** – Oxygen and circulation increase blood flow to all areas of the body, revitalizing your muscles throughout the entire day.

4. **Nervous System** – Keeps the spine flexible and the muscles around the vertebrae toned, balancing the nerves in the body.

5. **Digestive** – Proper nutrition is an important part of Yoga. Certain yoga postures stimulate the digestive tract.

6. **Elimination** – Stimulates peristalsis, and cleanses the digestive tract, blood, and skin. Yoga also helps flush out toxins in the body.

7. **Respiratory** – The lungs bring in oxygen and eliminate carbon dioxide. Poor concentration and mental fatigue can be caused by lack of oxygen. The deep breathing in Yoga cleanses the cardiovascular system.

8. **Glandular** – The glands regulate the body's metabolism and vital functions including mental state, energy level, and sexual drive. Certain poses help balance specific glands.

9. **Mental state** – A sound body requires a sound mind. Yoga helps produce mental clarity, concentration, and patience, in addition to releasing mental stress and fatigue. Self-observation and inquiry are important elements of Yoga.

10. **Spirit** – Yoga helps you achieve a calm, centered feeling while giving you renewed energy. It helps you turn your attention inward and reach a state of relaxation.

Some Basic Benefits of the Poses:

Standing Pose – Flexibility, strength, and stamina.
Seated Pose – A healthy back, poise, and reflection.
Forward Bends – Soothing and introspective.
Backbends – Posture and flexibility.
Inverted – Circulation and stress reduction.

KNOWING HOW YOUR BODY WORKS

To stimulate the correct formation of your bones, it is important to have a basic understanding of the body's structure and joints. This will improve stretching and help your body move in a more relaxed and natural way.

The body is designed along a central upright axis. The skull, rib cage, spine, and pelvis enclose and protect your vital organs. Your bones and limbs act as levers to move the body. The joints are held together by ligaments, which are tough and elastic. The bones serve as attachments for the ligaments and the tendons attach the muscles to the bone. Muscles of all shapes and sizes are located in layers around the skeletal structure giving the body support, volume, and shape.

The spinal column is the foundation of the body. All the nerves in your entire body branch out from the spinal cord located inside the vertebral column. Muscular tension collects around this area causing pain. By systematically stretching your spine in all directions, you can release tension and help keep your body properly aligned.

The body should be stretched in six basic ways – forward, backward, side to side, and twisting in both directions. When you stretch the spine one direction you want to be sure to counterstretch.

Pose/Counterpose

The concepts of expansion and contraction in Yoga are essential. This guarantees that you are balancing your muscles and your body. Backbends should be followed by forward bends, while side stretches and twists are performed on both sides of your body. Yoga is organized with passive movements following active movements to train your body to contract and release completely.

Dynamic/Static

Moving into and out of postures warms up the muscles to hold certain poses.

You are never completely still even in balance poses. The body is always adjusting itself in small ways. And of course, there's constant movement inside the body's muscles, nerves, and cells. In many exercises, you move from one posture to another, linking poses together. Then, there are postures you hold while you breathe.

GETTING STARTED

When you first begin, do not be frustrated if you struggle to learn the basic exercises and correct posture. You will soon notice your strength increase and your concentration improve. The more you practice Yoga, the faster you will see improvement in your flexibility. A healthy body is pliable and well-stretched as well as strong and toned.

Life can create many stresses, both mentally and physically. Lack of sleep, long hours at work, and everyday worries all can cause im-

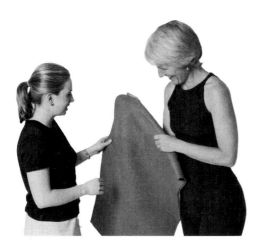

balance in your body. In addition, certain muscle groups are often overused during workouts. Yoga helps balance the nerves and muscles to prevent injury. Yoga can help diminish pain and aid the body's healing process.

By simultaneously activating numerous muscles in your body, Yoga facilitates correct alignment, detoxifies organs and tissues, and revitalizes the mind and body. Yoga increases the circulation of intercellular fluids, bringing in nutrients

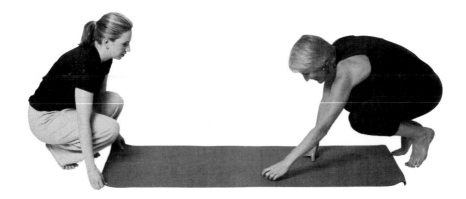

Before you begin:

1. Read through the entire book to become familiar with the poses.

2. Practice on an empty stomach.

3. Use a thin portable mat with a non-skid surface.

4. Wear comfortable clothes.

5. You can wear sneakers or go barefoot.

6. To help warm muscles, workout in a warm place with good ventilation.

7. Use a mirror only to check your posture. Your focus should be inward.

8. Consult with a doctor before beginning a yoga program if you are pregnant, recovering from an injury, or have never done Yoga before.

9. Practice in a quiet place where you will not be disturbed.

10. If you'd like, play soothing music to relax you while doing the poses.

while carrying off toxins.

In Yoga, we learn to pay attention to stress, releasing it from the body and mind. When a muscle is becoming tight, it is an indicator to do more Yoga. Because Yoga affects so many muscle groups, you will feel a tremendous difference at the finish of this workout. As you practice Yoga, you will develop the ability to sense pain and recognize which exercise will unlock discomfort. Tension in and around your joints often causes muscle stiffness. Practicing Yoga regularly can help release muscular tension.

Bodymind

Throughout this book, the words "body" and "mind" have been integrated to illustrated their union in Yoga as one entity. Mental stress is often reflected in your body as muscle spasms or thrown-off alignment. After a Yoga workout, you will feel balance in your muscles and revitalization in your mind.

BREATHING

Yoga integrates stretching and breathing. The bridge between our body and mind, breathing helps us concentrate on each pose. Breathing through the nose enables us to take fuller breaths. A person who has strong lungs and good breathing habits will most likely have more energy.

How we breathe can greatly affect our stress level and how we manage stress. We can use breathing as a tool to relax, clear our mind, and give us more energy. When you are nervous or anxious, you tend to breathe shallowly. When your mind is clear, you breathe evenly and fully. Often when we are learning a new pose, we have a tendency to hold our breath. Be sure to breathe throughout the entire exercise. Once you begin to integrate conscious breathing into Yoga, you will be able to take the poses further.

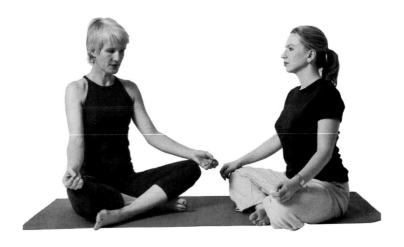

During the workout, emphasis is generally on the inhale to stimulate and energize. When a more passive or relaxed state is desired, the exhale is emphasized. Breathing through your nose helps to warm the body, making it easier to stretch. Pay attention to how you are breathing – be sure to breathe slowly and deeply.

There is a basic rule to remember for coordinating deep breathing with Yoga exercises. Inhale on the movement that is upward or expansive, and requires the most strength to stimulate. Exhale on the downward, folding and releasing movement, or when a more relaxed state is desired.

Hatha yoga coordinates deep breathing with the exercises using the diaphragm. The diaphragm is the muscle located in the abdominal area under the lungs, which extends down to the lowest rib. Before studying deep breathing, most people only use the top part of their lungs. Deep breathing techniques allow you to fill your entire lungs from the bottom to the top, improving your lung capacity. When you begin, don't worry about breathing correctly. The most important aspects to remember are to be sure not to hold your breath, and remember to inhale and exhale through your nose.

Part III: The Exercises

This pose will strengthen your back.

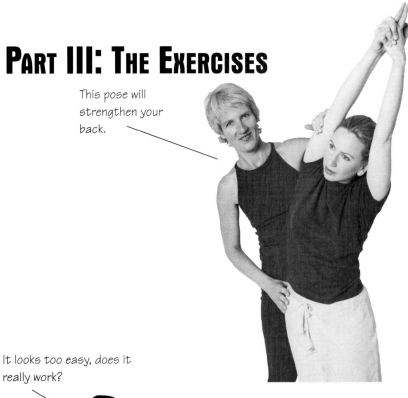

It looks too easy, does it really work?

You'll have powerful legs in no time with this stretch.

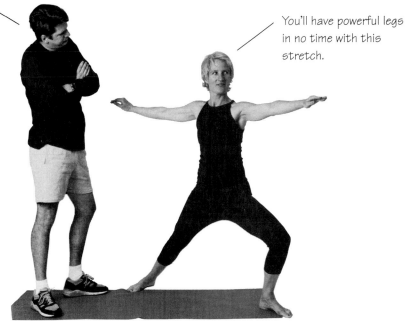

THE EXERCISES

Yoga is structured in a progression that allows you to increase the range of motion gradually. When you first learn a Yoga pose, it is just a technique. As you practice the exercise, it becomes more refined, smooth, and graceful. Always be attentive to your body when you are practicing Yoga. *Practice Yoga slowly. It is better to do fewer exercises than to rush.* Let the body stretch as far as it wants to go, then breathe and take it a little further.

Stretch to the point where you feel some degree of both pain and pleasure. If you only feel pain, you are pushing yourself too far. Re-

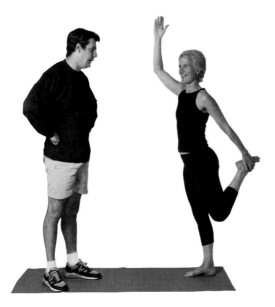

lease a little and focus on breathing. Imagine breathing in and out of a painful stretch. Long and full breaths are the keys to opening up tightness in the nerves and muscles. Be sure to remember that we are all individuals with different needs and abilities. Do not compare your flexibility to that of others. There is no competition in Yoga.

Keep in mind the union that balances the right and left sides of your body. Perform each exercise on both sides. Have a towel on hand to sit on and stretch with throughout your workout. Move slowly between exercises, taking each stretch further as your muscles continue to warm-up.

Sometimes after doing Yoga, you may feel light-headed or feel new sensations in your body. This is the result of an increase in circulation, which helps you to be more aware of your posture and breathing throughout the day.

Be sure to take the time to learn some of the basic stances and poses before you begin. Many of these positions are repeated throughout the workout as the foundation for more advanced poses.

Yoga Basics

Cross-Legged Seated Position – Sit in a comfortable position with your legs crossed in front of you. Resting on your sit bones, drop your shoulders and lift your stomach, chest, and head. Take full-breaths in and out of nose, counting to three as you inhale and exhale.

Benefit: warms up hip sockets, encourages correct breathing, and improves posture.

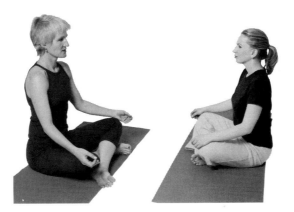

Cross-Legged Seated Position

Note:
The sit bones refer to the bottom of your hip girdle as shown in Illustration A.

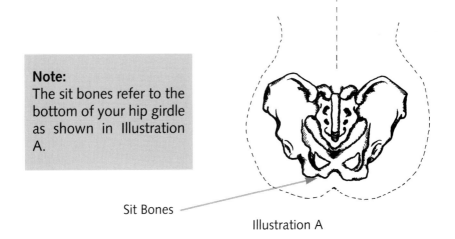

Sit Bones

Illustration A

Three Part Breath – Although conscious breathing is integrated into all the poses in Yoga, this is the most basic breathing exercise. Inhale through your nose for a count of three, and hold for another count of three before exhaling. Breathing through the nose is important because it encourages us to take full and deep breaths.

Benefit: demonstrates full breathing, and increases circulation in the torso muscles.

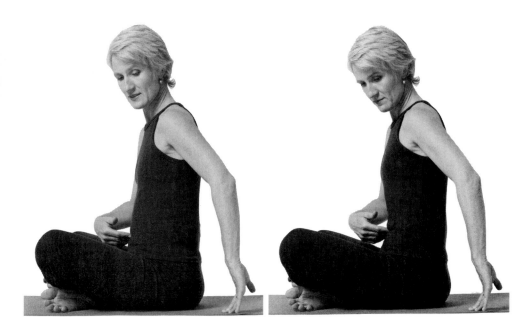

Three Part Breath

Mountain Pose – With your feet planted on the floor, use your leg muscles to stack your body – feet, knees, hips, and rib cage. Widen your chest, drop your shoulders, and feel your neck and back of head lengthen.

Benefit: helps alignment and balance, releases shoulders, and lengthens neck.

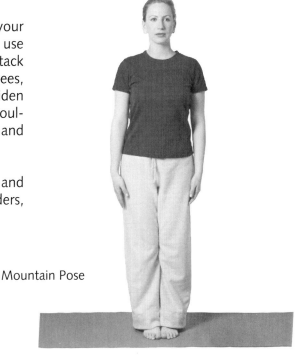

Mountain Pose

Note:
Yoga will teach you to maintain alignment of the spine and joints. Stacking refers to the basic mountain pose. The ankle, knee, hip, shoulder, and ear lobe are all vertically lined up. This is called the plum line. See Illustration B.

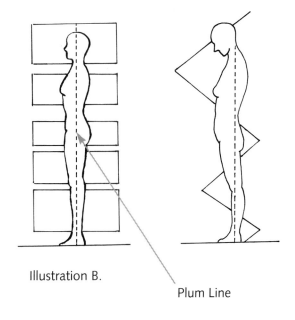

Illustration B.

Plum Line

Mountain Pose Variation – Interlace your fingers and raise your arms above you. Straighten your arms, keeping them close to your head. Repeat three times.

Benefit: helps to lengthen the back, releases tension between the shoulders, and increases circulation to the head.

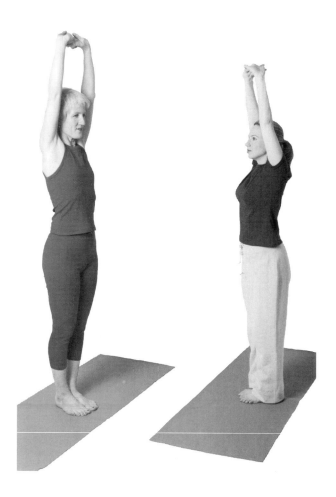

Mountain Pose Variation

Standing Forward Bend

Standing Forward Bend – Roll your head down slowly, hang forward, and release your neck. Reach your sit bones up as you drop your head forward.

Benefit: increases flexibility of the spine, sciatic nerve, and most of the tendons and ligaments in the legs; firms and trims the waist, buttocks, and thighs; and improves circulation to the legs, back, and brain.

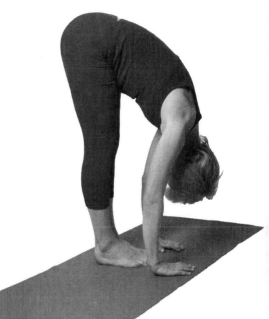

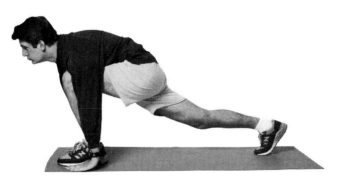

Lunge

Lunge – From a standing forward bend, drop your right foot approximately four feet behind you. Keep your left knee bent over your left toes and lengthen your neck. Focus on a point on the ground ahead of you as you lift your stomach muscles.

Benefit: stretches the quadriceps, limbers the hips, tightens the buttocks, and encourages correct positioning of the knees.

Triangle Pose – With your feet three to four feet apart, turn your left foot out slightly and line up your right heel with your left ankle. Place your arms by your hips or stretched out to the sides parallel to the floor. Remember to lift your knees to engage the thighs.

Benefit: works and tones the calves, thighs and hamstrings.

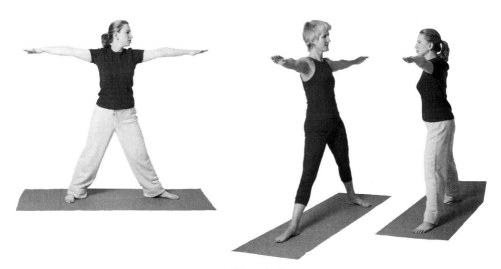

Triangle Pose

Child Pose – On your knees, release your pelvis and drop your butt to your heels. Stretch your arms out in front of you and lower your head to the ground. This is a basic relaxation pose to do if you are tired between exercises.

Benefit: releases back muscles.

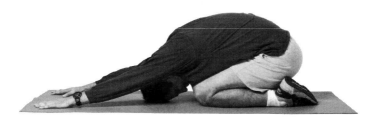

Child Pose

BEGINNING STRETCHES

Seated Side Stretch – Sit in the basic Cross-Legged position with your sit bones planted on the ground. Placing your left hand on the floor, stretch your right arm over your head close to your ear. Return back to center and repeat with your opposite arm. Perform three times on either side.

Benefit: tones stomach and torso muscles, and stretches the back.

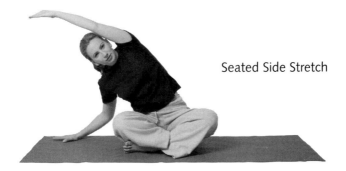

Seated Side Stretch

Seated Forward Stretch – Sitting in the Cross-Legged position, stretch forward, drop your head, and lean into both hands while you breathe. Repeat twice.

Benefit: warms up the back muscles and releases lower back tension.

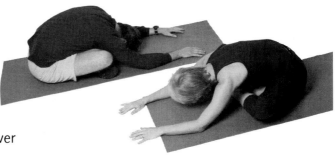

Seated Forward Stretch

23

Seated Hamstring Stretch – With your legs together, rest on your sit bones as you lift your arms up overhead and stretch forward to your toes or shins. Make sure your knees are facing upwards. Bend your knees slightly if you cannot reach your toes or use a towel held beneath your feet. Inhale as you look forward. Exhale as you bend your elbows and reach your chest toward your thighs. Take three full breaths.

Benefit: Improves digestion, helps balance blood sugar level, and improves flexibility of the Sciatic nerves, ankles, knees, and hip joints.

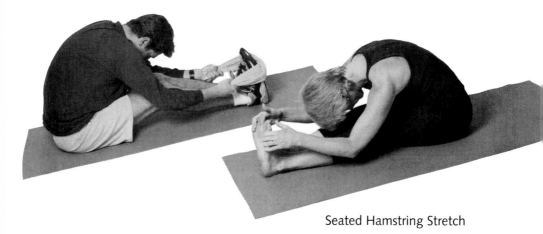

Seated Hamstring Stretch

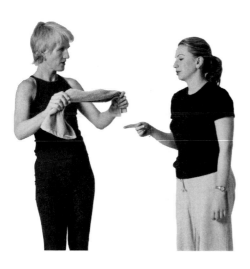

Note: Hold a small towel around your foot for additional flexibility.

Cat Pose – On your hand and knees, place your hands under your shoulders and your knees under your hips. Arch and round your back. Integrate breathing by inhaling as you arch and exhaling as you round.

Benefit: lengthens the back, and warms the muscles, spine, and digestive organs.

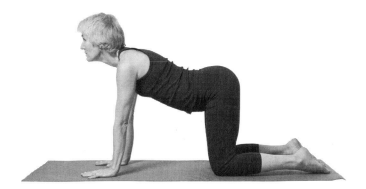

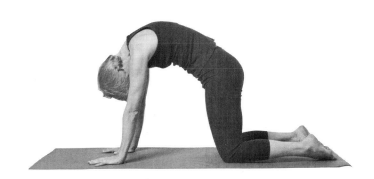

Cat Pose

Runner's Lunge – Place your left foot forward and your right leg back. Put your hands beside your left foot and straighten your right leg. Bend and drop your right leg and repeat.

Benefit: warms up your quadriceps and tightens the butt muscles.

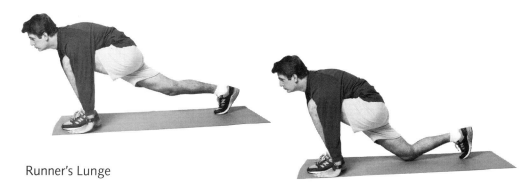

Runner's Lunge

Runner's Lunge Variation – With both feet together facing forward, drop your left leg three to four feet behind you. Straighten your right leg as much as you can while you flex and release your right foot three times. Repeat on the both sides.

Benefit: releases the lower back, increases circulation to the hip sockets, and stretches the hamstrings and Achilles tendon.

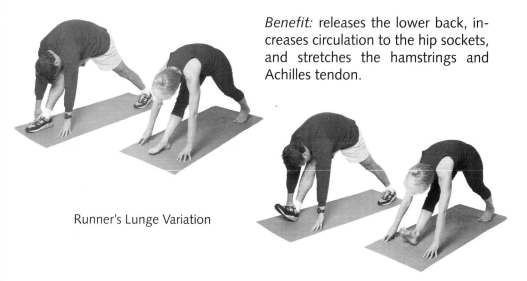

Runner's Lunge Variation

Down Dog – Press your hands and feet into the floor and lift your hips high in the air. Lengthen the back muscles up towards your hip sockets and release your butt muscles. Bend and straighten your knees three times to slowly open the hamstrings. Straighten your legs and hold the pose for six long breaths.

Benefit: releases lower back, and strengthens upper back and hamstring muscles.

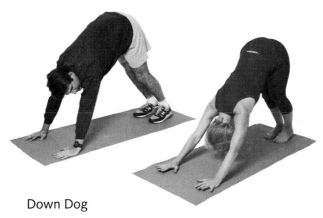

Down Dog

Down Dog Leg Stretch – From the Down Dog position, raise your right leg in the air and bend your knee. Pull your right heel to your left buttocks and repeat with your left leg.

Benefit: stretches and releases the hip socket, opens the front of the hip, and strengthens the shoulders.

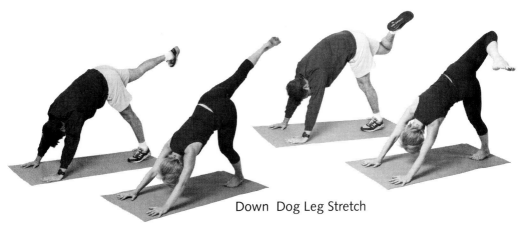

Down Dog Leg Stretch

Plank Pose – Bring your body parallel to the ground. Tighten your butt and abdominal muscles as you stretch your arms out straight. Lengthen the back and look straight down.

Benefit: serves as a good transition pose and strengthens the abs, shoulders, and mid-back.

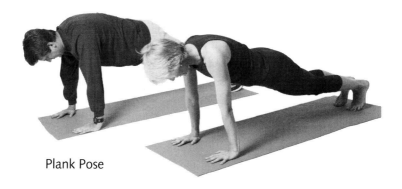

Plank Pose

Plank Pose Variation – From the Plank Pose, drop your knees, chest, and chin down to the mat.

Benefit: important transition exercise, strengthens the lumbar section of the back and the abdominal muscles.

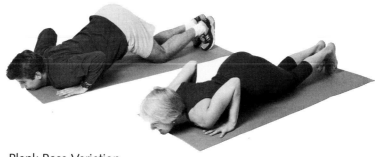

Plank Pose Variation

Reverse Push-up – From the Plank Pose, bend your arms with your elbows close to your sides, keeping your body straight. Slowly lower your body and repeat.

Benefit: strengthens the abdominal muscles, and tones the chest and arms.

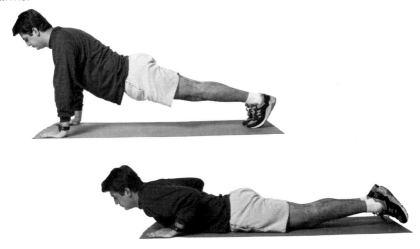

Reverse Push-up

Up Dog – From the Plank Pose, slowly bend your elbows and swing your hips forward to your hands with your knees and feet on the ground. If your back is strong enough, lift your knees off the ground.

Benefit: strengthens arms and shoulders, and tones the digestive and reproductive systems.

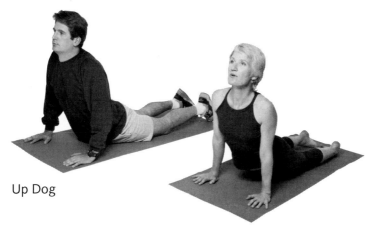

Up Dog

29

Standing Swimmer's Stretch – Starting from the Mountain Pose position, keep your arms straight and interlace your fingers behind you as you drop your head to your knees.

Benefit: releases tension in the back, helps prevent rotator cuff injuries, and improves the range of shoulder motion.

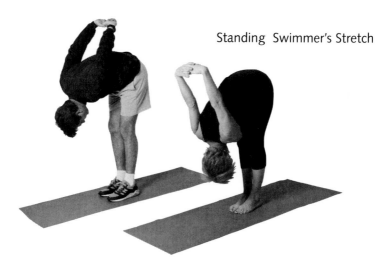

Standing Swimmer's Stretch

Roll Up – As you stand in the Forward Bend position with your fingers touching the floor, roll your back and head up and down slowly. Inhale as you roll up and exhale as you roll back down. Repeat three times.

Benefit: overall relaxation.

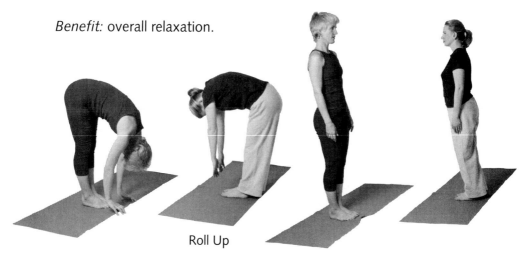

Roll Up

Half Moon – Lift your arms overhead with your palms together. Reach your arms to one side. Slowly return back to center. Lift your torso from the hips and line up your head and arms. Tighten your buttocks, lift your stomach for three full breaths, and repeat on the other side. Release to the Mountain Pose.

Benefit: gives you energy, strengthens the muscles in your torso and back, and increases flexibility in the spine, correcting bad posture.

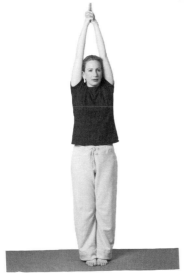

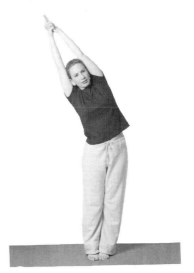

Half Moon

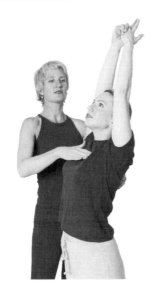

Half Moon Variation

Half Moon Variation – From the Mountain Pose, bring your palms together above your head and point your index fingers. Arch your back and lift your chest. Return to the Mountain Pose and roll forward.

Benefit: releases tension between the shoulder blades, expands the chest, and helps to correct posture and round the upper back.

31

Triangle Side Stretch – Assume the Triangle Pose and tilt back from the tailbone, moving your entire back and not just your waist. Slide your right hand down your right shin and stretch your left arm to the sky.

Benefit: tones the waist, hips, thighs, and backs of legs, and promotes balance.

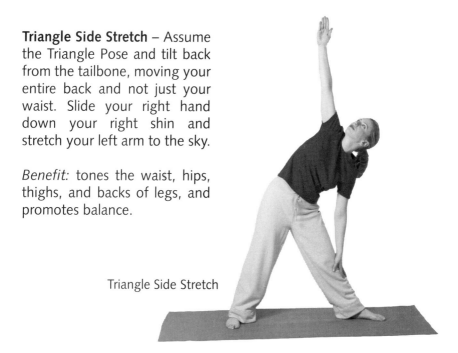

Triangle Side Stretch

Proud Warrior – From the Triangle Pose, bend your knee while keeping your thigh parallel to the ground. With your palms down, lift your arms out to the sides and look out towards the tips of your fingers. Hold the pose for a count of ten and repeat on the other side.

Benefit: strengthens legs and helps the alignment of the back.

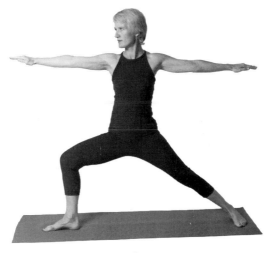

Proud Warrior

Dancer Pose – With your left foot on the ground, reach your left arm up and hold your right leg behind you while focusing on a point in front of you. If necessary, use a wall or chair to help you balance initially. Hold for a count of ten. Repeat on the other side.

Benefit: increases concentration and stretches the front of your thigh.

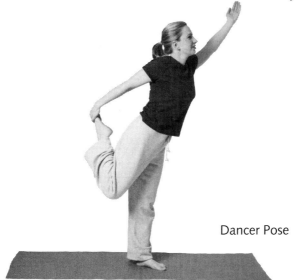

Dancer Pose

Pelvic Tilt – Lie on your back and bend your knees. Tighten your butt muscles as you slowly lift your back until you feel the weight across your shoulders. Stop at the base of your neck and hold for a count of three breaths. Clasp your hands under your hips as you hold the pose.

Benefit: strengthens and tightens your butt muscles, increases circulation in your back and hips, and relaxes the entire nervous system.

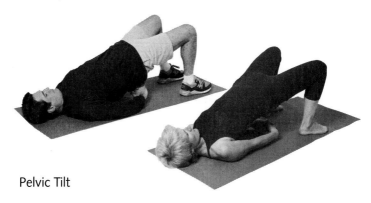

Pelvic Tilt

Yoga Sit-up – Lie on your back with your knees bent and your feet flat on the ground as you inhale. Cradle your head with your hands and exhale as you lift your head and upper body. Feel your abdominal muscles tighten as you lift your head slightly towards your knees.

Benefit: tones all stomach muscles.

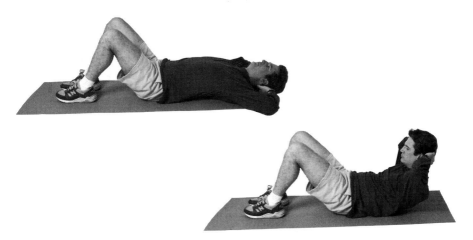

Yoga Sit-up

Twisted Yoga Sit-up – Lie on your back with both knees bent and your feet on the floor. Rest your left calf over your right thigh. Interlace your fingers behind your head as you inhale. Bring your right elbow to your left knee as you exhale. Repeat several times and switch sides.

Benefit: works all the stomach muscles, including the internal and external obliques.

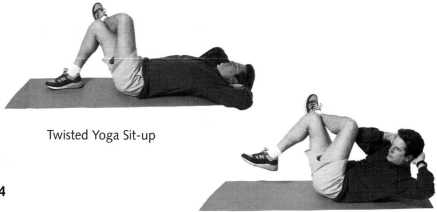

Twisted Yoga Sit-up

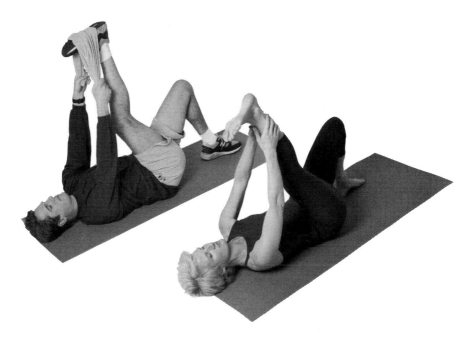

Hamstring Stretch

Hamstring Stretch – Laying on your back, leave one leg on the ground and straighten one leg into the air. Hold onto a towel or your calf and point and flex your toes three times.

Benefit: stretches the hamstring and calf muscles.

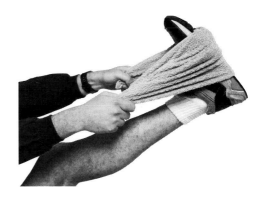

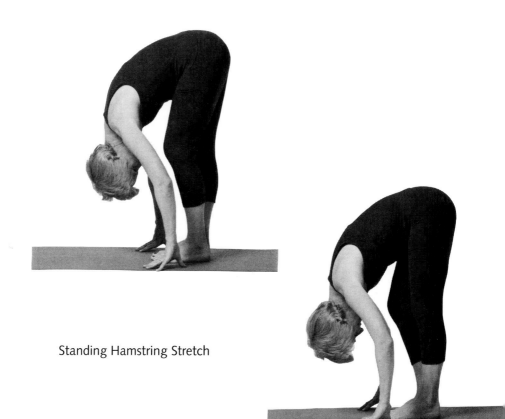

Standing Hamstring Stretch

Standing Hamstring Stretch – Arch your upper back and roll forward. Relax your back, soften your abdominal muscles, and tighten your hamstrings. With your feet slightly apart, bend one knee while keeping the other one straight. Repeat three times on each side.

Benefit: warms up hamstrings and releases lower back tension.

Butterfly – Sitting on your hip sockets with the soles of your feet together and your knees out to the sides, stretch your head down to your toes.

Benefit: opens hip sockets, and releases lower back, inner thighs, and sacrum.

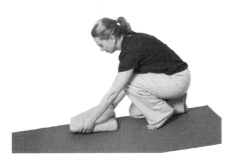
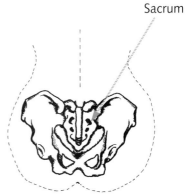

Butterfly

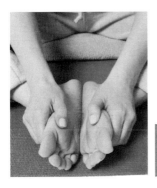

Note: A towel can also be used under your sit bones for additional flexibility.

Sacrum

Note:
Sacrum – A triangular bone situated at the bottom of the vertebrae. Its articulation forms the Sacroiliac joint. See Illustration A.

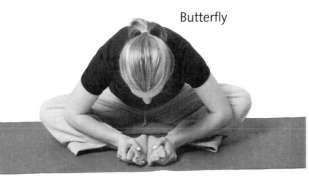

Illustration A

Modified Hurdler – Bring your right foot into your left thigh and straighten your left leg. Exhale as you stretch towards your straightened leg, and inhale as you return back. Try to stretch further down your leg with each exhale. Hold your position,take three full breaths, and repeat on the opposite side.

Benefit: prevents sciatica and limbers up the ankles, knees, and hip sockets.

Note:
Sciatica – Severe pain in the leg along the course of the sciatic nerve. It is felt at the back of the thigh and runs down the back of the leg.

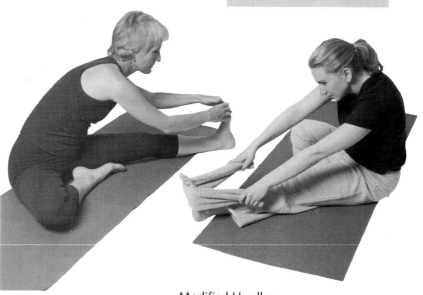

Modified Hurdler

Shoulder Rolls- Roll your shoulders up, back, and around three times in each direction.

Benefit: releases shoulder tension and improves posture.

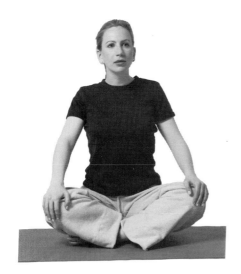

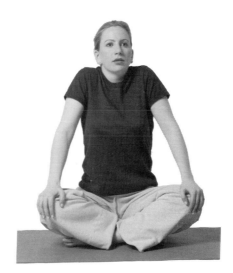

Shoulder Rolls

Neck Rolls – Stretch your left ear towards your left shoulder and then your right ear towards your right shoulder. Roll your head left, forward, and to the right. Inhale as you roll your head to each side, and exhale as your roll your head forward. Be careful not to crunch your neck back.

Benefit: releases tension in the neck and increases circulation to the brain.

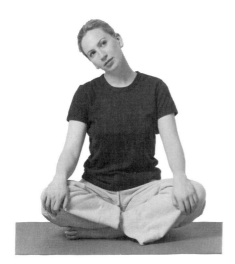

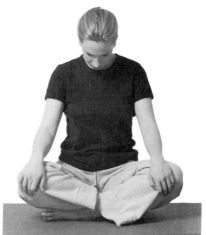

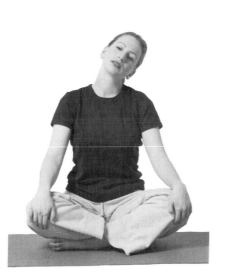

ADVANCED STRETCHES

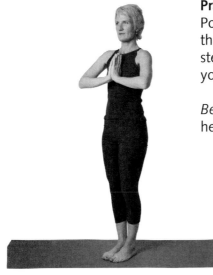

Prayer Pose – From the Mountain Pose, bring your palms together in the middle of your chest along your sternum, paying close attention to your breathing.

Benefit: good transition pose and helps to center the Bodymind.

Prayer Pose

Prayer Pose Squat – From the Prayer Pose, bend your knees as far as you can, keeping your legs together and your back straight.

Benefit: lengthens the back, and strengthens the buttocks and thigh muscles.

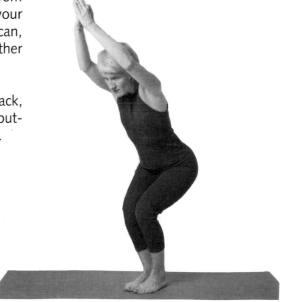

Prayer Pose Squat

41

Prayer Pose Squat Variation – From the Prayer Pose Squat position, twist your body to the left and press your right elbow against the outside of the left leg. Repeat on the left side.

Benefit: balances the nervous system, tones the waist, and enhances digestion.

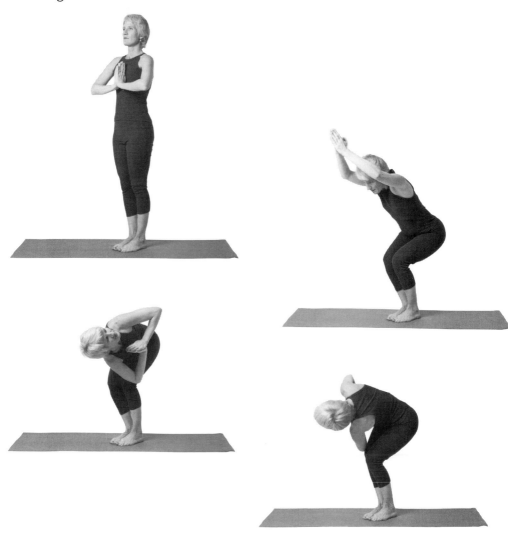

Prayer Pose Squat Variation

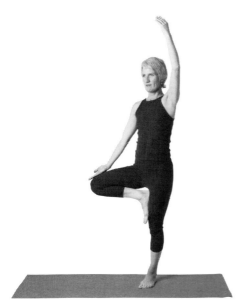

Tree Balance – Stand on your left leg and lift your right foot onto your left ankle and eventually up to the inside of your left thigh. Raise your left arm up and place your right hand on your right knee for balance. Count three breaths and repeat on the other side.

Benefit: increases balance and mental concentration, and strengthens leg muscles and torso.

Tree Balance

Warrior Side Stretch – From the triangle pose, stand with your feet apart and bend your left knee. Lean your left forearm on your left thigh. Stretch your right arm over your head, close to your ear. Return to the Down Dog position and repeat this pose on the other side of your body. Remember to breathe in and out through your nose.

Benefit: improves balance and respiration, stretches both sides of the body, and releases tension in the shoulders.

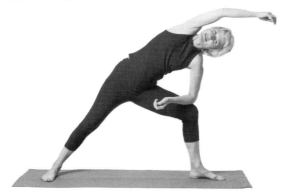

Warrior Side Stretch

43

Standing Spinal Twist – Standing in the triangle pose with your right leg back, lift in your arms parallel to the ground. Bend from the hip sockets as you twist your torso, reaching your right arm down your left leg and stretching your left arm towards the sky. Breathe, return to the Down Dog position, and repeat on the other side.

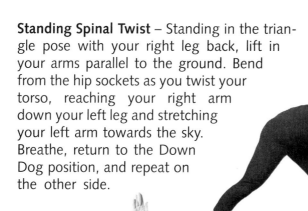

Benefit: stimulates the internal organs, helps balance the nervous system, and increases flexibility and tone in the back.

Standing Spinal Twist

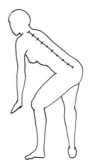

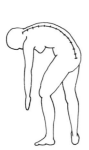

Incorrect

Bending from the Hips

Illustration D.

Note: In Yoga, it is important to bend from the hip sockets and not the back, which can put unnecessary stress on your spine and back muscles, increasing the chance of injury. Bending from the hips releases tightness around the hip sockets while toning surrounding muscles. See Illustration D.

Camel Pose – While on your knees, flex your feet and align your pelvis over your knees. Arch your torso and reach your right hand down to the right heel, and your left arm over your head. Switch sides and repeat with your left hand. Take full breaths as you arch your body and reach both your hands and your head back in a comfortable position.

Benefit: helps to cure constipation, good for respiration, trims the waistline, and balances strength and flexibility in the torso.

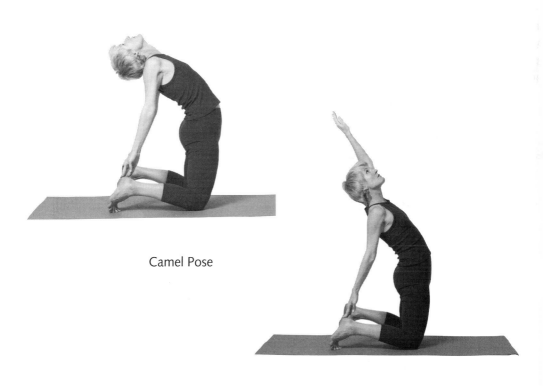

Camel Pose

Seated Spinal Twist – Rest on your sit bones with both legs out in front of you. Bend your right leg over your left leg as you reach your right arm behind you and your left arm against the outside of your right thigh. Twist from your pelvis through your lower, middle, and upper back, including the neck. Twist, lift, and breathe before gently releasing to the left. Repeat on the opposite side.

Benefit: rejuvenates the nervous system and increases flexibility in the spine.

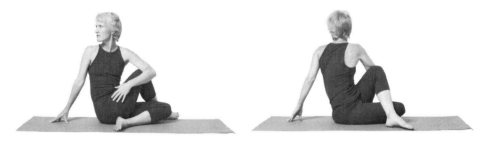

Seated Spinal Twist

Breath of Fire – Sit cross-legged and start with a series of Three Part Breaths. Elevate yourself slightly off the ground and soften your lower abdominals. Take smaller breaths, quickly inhaling and exhaling as your stomach muscles contract. Repeat this exercise twenty times.

Benefit: tones internal organs and abdominal muscles.

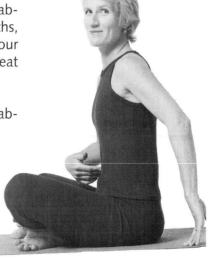

Breath of Fire

Inner Thigh Stretch – Rest on your sit bones with your legs spread apart. Stretch your hands out on the floor in front of you and release your neck. Keep your back straight and release your stomach muscles. Place a towel under your sit bones or bend your knees slightly if have difficulty stretching forward. This exercise can also be done with a partner.

Benefit: relaxes the lower back and hip sockets, and stretches the inner thigh muscles.

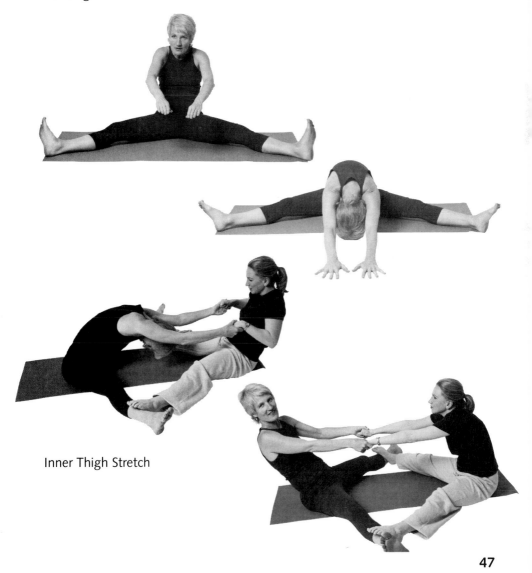

Inner Thigh Stretch

Superman pose – Laying on your stomach, release all your weight into the ground and tune into your breathing. With your legs and hips planted, and your arms over your head, inhale. Exhale as you lift your head, shoulders, and feet off the ground. Keep your feet to-gether and hold this pose for a count of three and release.

Benefit: strengthens the back muscles, especially the Erector Spine.

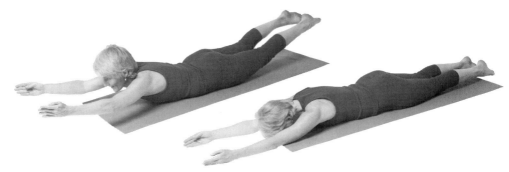

Superman pose

Superman #2 – From the Superman pose, reach your arms behind you. Raise your upper body and feet off the ground. Hold for three breaths, lift slightly higher, and release your head to the side.

Benefit: strengthens the lower back and pelvic organs, and releases tension from the shoulders and between the shoulder blades.

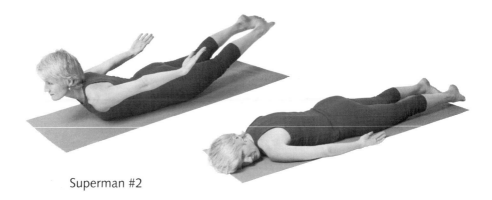

Superman #2

Bow – Lie on your stomach and bend your knees. Reach your hands back and hold your ankles. Focus on a point in front of you and incorporate your breath by inhaling as you rock back and exhaling as you rock forward. Try to hold this pose for six full breaths.

Benefit: increases flexibility in the back, tones abdominal wall, releases tension, and improves digestion.

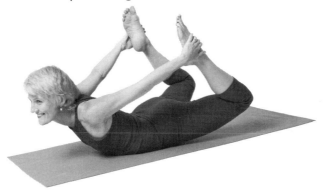

Bow

Cobra – Lie on your stomach with your hands directly under your shoulders. Breathe in and exhale as you lift your head, upper back, and stomach off the ground. Slowly release your chin as you relax back into the ground.

Benefit: Strengthens the upper back and stimulates internal organs.

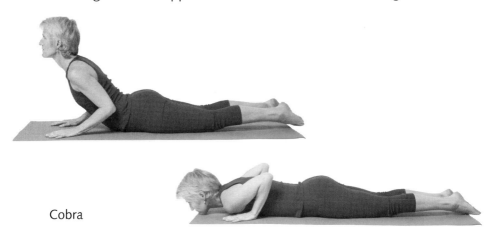

Cobra

Spinal Roll – Lie on your back and hug your legs in against your chest. Roll back and forth on your spine, breathing gently. Roll back into the sitting position.

Benefit: massages the muscles of the back, helps balance the nervous system, and functions as a good transition pose.

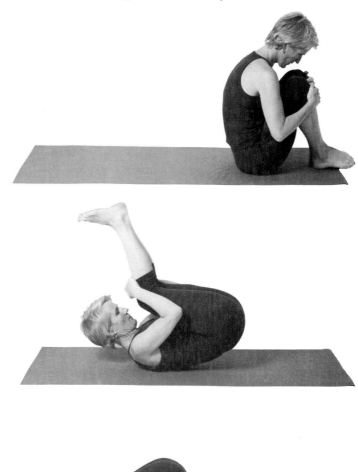

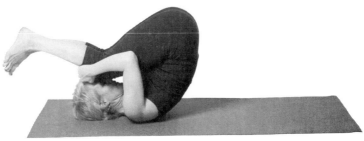

Spinal Roll

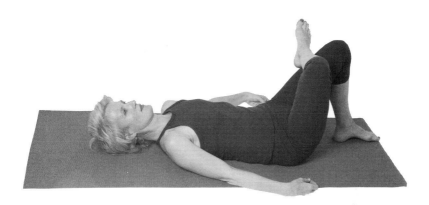

Hip Socket Stretch

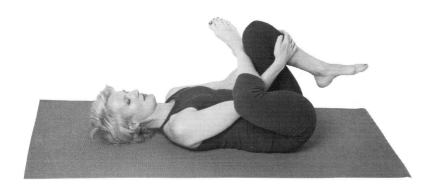

Hip Socket Stretch – Lie on your back with your knees bent. Cross your right calf over your left thigh, twisting from the hip. Wrap your hands around your left hamstring or shin and gently pull towards you. Breathe and repeat on the other side.

Benefit: increases circulation and toning around the hip.

51

Boat Pose – Balance on your sit bones and straighten your legs as much possible. Hold your arms out in front of you for balance. Hold the pose for a count of ten and repeat.

Benefit: tones your stomach muscles.

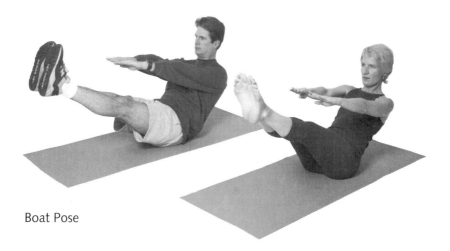

Boat Pose

Boat Pose Variation – From the Boat Pose position, bend your knees slightly to the right and lift onto your left sit bones for a count of ten. Shift your body and repeat on your right sit bones. Hold your arms out to the opposite side you are shifting for additional balance.

Benefit: tones the obliques, and trims the waist and lower ab-domen.

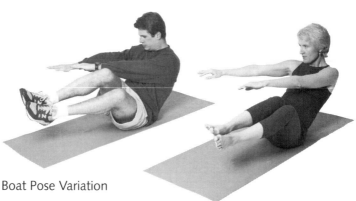

Boat Pose Variation

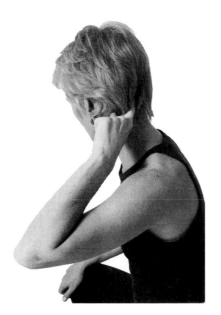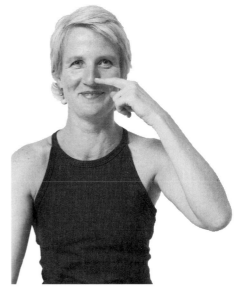

Head Rolls

Head Rolls – Sit cross-legged with your hands on your lap. Keep your neck still as you rotate your head. Outline the movement with the tip of your nose, moving it clockwise and counterclockwise three times in each direction.

Benefit: reduces eye strain, invigorates the mind, and reduces tension headaches.

Plow – From a sitting position, slowly roll your legs up over your head onto the floor behind you. Bend your knees towards your shoulder and release. Clasp your arms behind you.

Benefit: conditions the nervous and the endocrine systems.

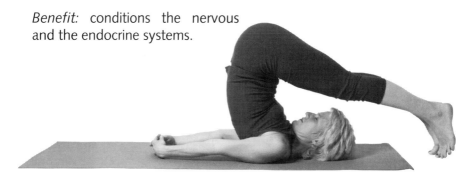

Plow

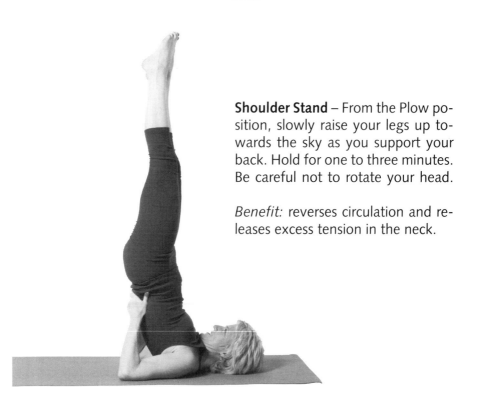

Shoulder Stand – From the Plow position, slowly raise your legs up towards the sky as you support your back. Hold for one to three minutes. Be careful not to rotate your head.

Benefit: reverses circulation and releases excess tension in the neck.

Shoulder Stand

Fish Pose – Lying on your back, bring your feet and legs together and relax. Lift your body up on your elbows and arch your back from your tailbone to your neck and hold.

Benefit: balances the back and nerves after doing Shoulder Stands.

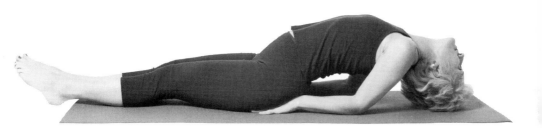

Fish Pose

SPECIFIC TARGET AREAS

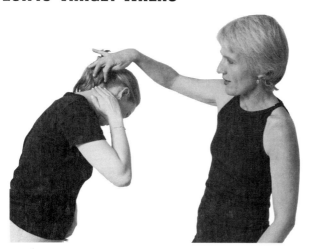

Why is it important to do specific target area exercises? All our bodies have certain strengths and weaknesses. Since Yoga focuses on balance, we need to target our areas of weakness and strengthen them by doing specific Yoga exercises.

By performing target area exercises three times a week, you can effectively reduce strain, and strengthen muscles in weak areas. They can also be combined with the sequences in Part IV to create complete workouts. Focus in on muscle groups to feel and see results.

Lower Back

Mountain Pose – helps alignment and balance, releases shoulders, and lengthens neck.

Standing Forward Bend – increases flexibility of the spine, sciatic nerve, and most of the tendons and ligaments in the legs; and improves circulation to the legs, back, and brain.

Proud Warrior – helps alignment of the back, and releases tightness in the sacrum region.

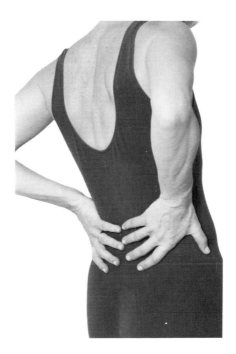

Cat Pose – lengthens the back, and warms up the muscles and spine.

Cobra – increases spinal strength and flexibility, and helps prevent lower backache.

Down Dog – releases the lower back and strengthens the upper back.

Child Pose – releases all back muscles.

Hamstring Stretch – releases lower back tension.

Pelvic Tilt – increases circulation in the back and hips.

Yoga Sit-up – tones all stomach muscles, and encourages correct integrated breathing.

Butterfly – opens hip sockets, releases lower back, inner thighs, and sacrum.

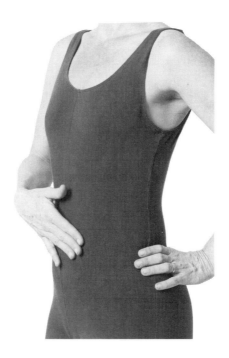

Stomach Strengthening Poses

Strong abdominal muscles are essential for good posture, coordination, and balance, engaging your abdominal muscles to help support and protect your back. There are four major abdominal groups:

1. *Rectus Abdominals* – attaching from the pubic bone to the center of the torso.

2. *Transverse Abdominals* – wrapping around the spine.

3. *Internal Oblique* – inner layer of muscles running from the lower ribs to the lower abdomen in a V-shape formation.

4. *External Oblique* – outer layer of muscles running from the lower ribs to the lower abdomen in a V-shape formation.

Three Part Breath – shows how to breathe fully, increases circulation in the torso, and tones the transverse muscles.

Breath of Fire – tones the internal organs and the rectus abdominals.

Yoga Sit-up – tones all stomach muscles, and encourages correct abdominal breathing.

Twisted Yoga Sit-up – works all the stomach muscles, including the internal and external obliques.

Boat Pose – isometric for the obliques, and allows the stomach to use a full range of muscle, contracting and releasing completely.

Boat Pose Variation – tones the obliques, trims the waist, and strengthens the lower abdominal muscles.

Butterfly – opens hip sockets and releases lower back.

Cat Pose – lengthens your back, and warms up the muscles and spine.

Bow Pose – increases flexibility in the back, tones abdominal wall, and releases tension.

Posture Check Poses

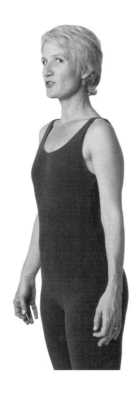
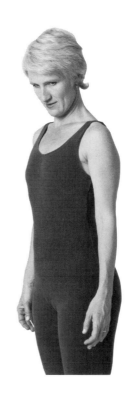

Note:
Posture check poses
stack the body from
the feet up.
See Illustration B.

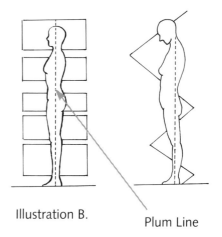

Illustration B.

Plum Line

Mountain Pose – helps alignment and balance, releases the shoulders, and lengthens the neck.

Half Moon – gives you energy, strengthens muscles in the torso and back, and increases flexibility in the spine, correcting bad posture.

Half Moon Variation – releases tension between the shoulder blades, expands the chest, and helps to round the upper back and correct posture.

Standing Hamstring Stretch – releases lower back tension.

Proud Warrior – helps alignment of the back.

Cross-legged Seated Position – warms up hip sockets, encourages correct breathing, and improves posture.

Upper Back and Neck Strengthening Exercises

The upper back and neck are common areas for tension and discomfort. We can stretch and strengthen these areas to help prevent injury. Tension does not collect in a strong, balanced muscle, having complete range to fully tighten and release. Tension likes to hide in malfunctioning and imbalanced muscles groups.

Movements of the head should originate where the base of the head meets the top of the neck, a unique joint composed of the top two vertebrae. This joint allows great freedom of motion to turn, lift, nod and rotate your head. Movement of the neck should originate from the seventh cervical. (see Illustration E).

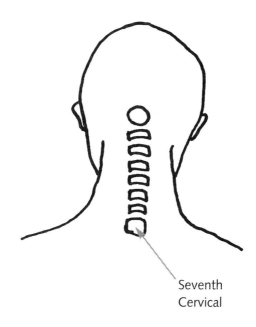

Seventh
Cervical

Illustration E.

Standing Swimmer's Stretch – releases tension in the back, helps prevent rotator cuff injuries, and improves the range of shoulder motion.

Dancer Pose – increases concentration and flexibility in the upper back and shoulders.

Half Moon – gives you energy, strengthens muscles in the torso and back, and increases flexibility in the spine.

Spinal Roll – massages the muscles of the back and functions as a good transition pose.

Cobra Pose – strengthens upper back muscles.

Seated Spinal Twist – increases flexibility in your spine.

Neck Rolls – releases tension in the neck and shoulders.

Head Rolls – increases mobility in the neck and reduces tension.

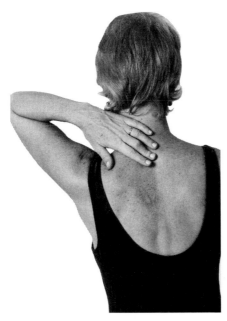

Chest and Upper Arms

Down Dog – strengthens the pectoral and deltoid muscles.

Plank Pose – tones the chest and arms.

Up Dog – stretches the chest leading to improved use of the chest and arm muscles.

Reverse Push-up – good transition pose that uses the chest, arms, and upper back.

Camel – stretches the chest and deltoid muscles.

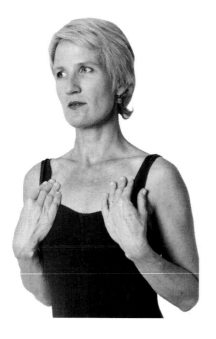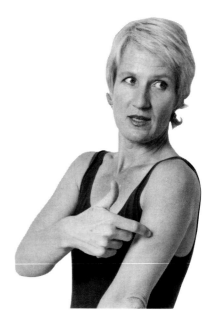

PART IV: THE WORKOUTS

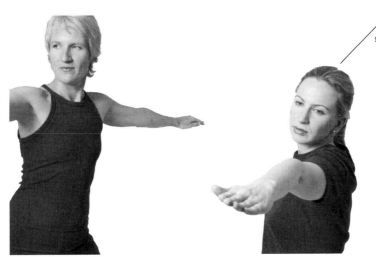

I am really starting to feel good.

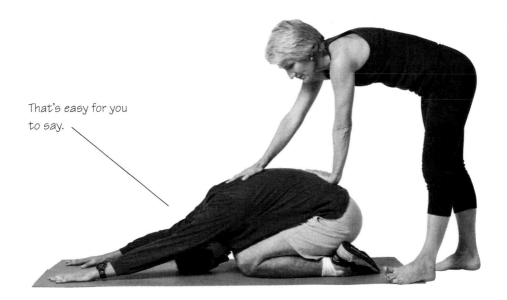

That's easy for you to say.

SALUTATIONS

Sun salutations are perfectly balanced yoga progressions. Salutations stretch almost every major muscle group in your body. They incorporate balance, forward bending, backward bending, and neutral exercises. These routines enhance strength and flexibility.

Salutations warm up the muscles quickly and can be done with your ten-minute sequences or longer variations. The Sun Salutations are designed to flow from one position to the next. It is important to remember to breathe fully, and not to hold your breath. When you first begin, focus on learning the saluation and the breathing. As you become more familiar with the salutations, you will begin to inhale and exhale with each pose.

SUN SALUTATION #1

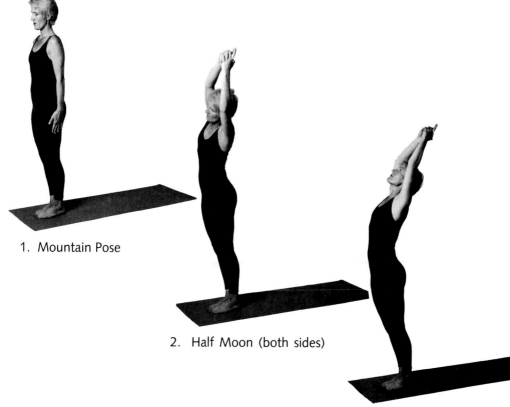

1. Mountain Pose

2. Half Moon (both sides)

3. Half Moon Variation

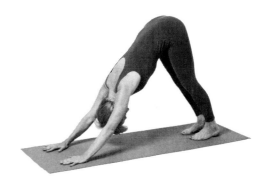

6. Down Dog

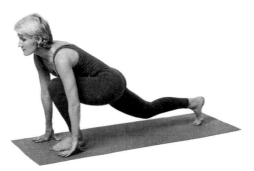

5. Lunge, right leg back

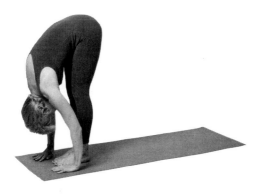

4. Standing Forward Bend

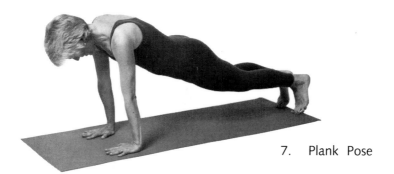

7.   Plank   Pose

8. Up Dog

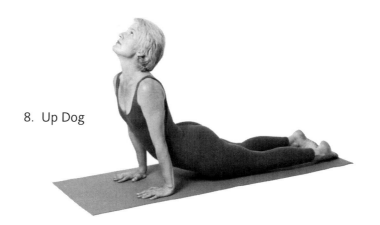

9. Down Dog

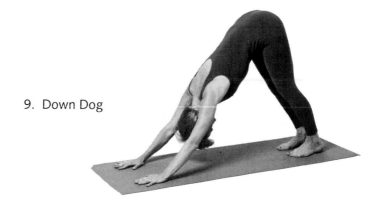

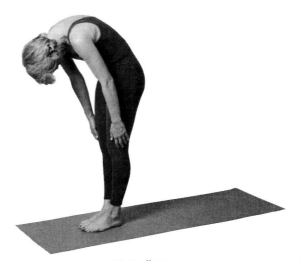

12. Roll Up

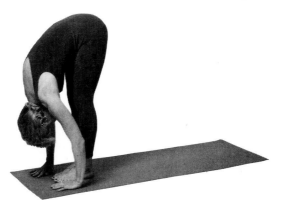

11. Standing Forward Bend

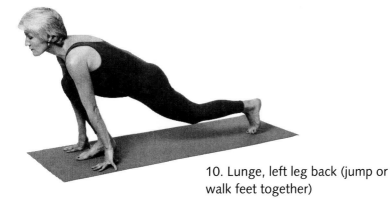

10. Lunge, left leg back (jump or
walk feet together)

SUN SALUTATION #2

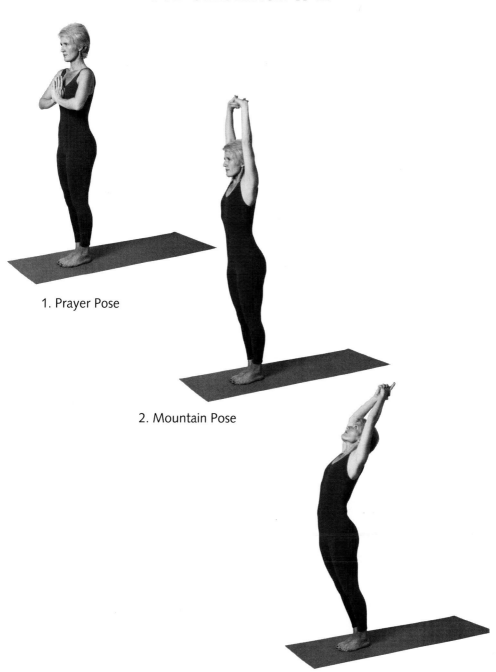

1. Prayer Pose

2. Mountain Pose

3. Half Moon Variation

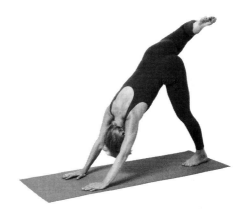

6. Down Dog Leg Stretch (both sides)

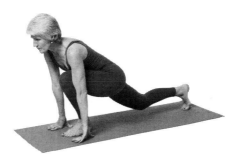

5. Lunge, right leg back

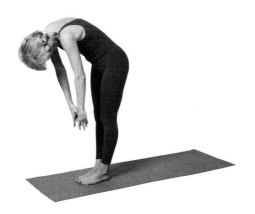

4. Roll Down

71

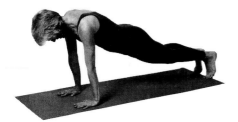

7. Plank Pose

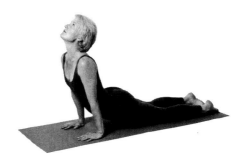

8. Up Dog

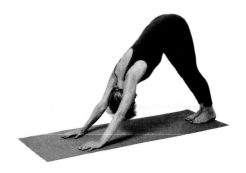

9. Down Dog

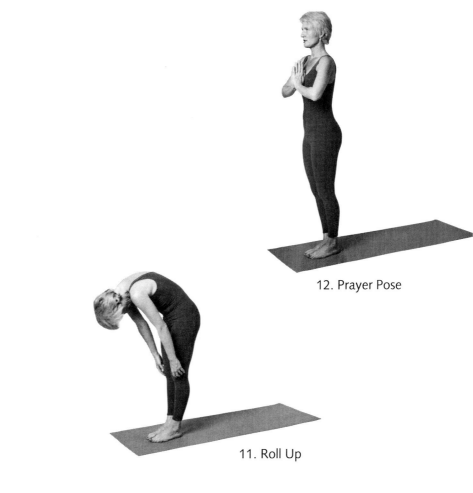

12. Prayer Pose

11. Roll Up

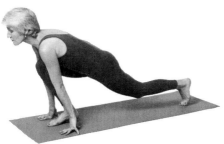

10. Lunge, left leg back (jump or walk feet together)

73

SUN SALUTATION #3

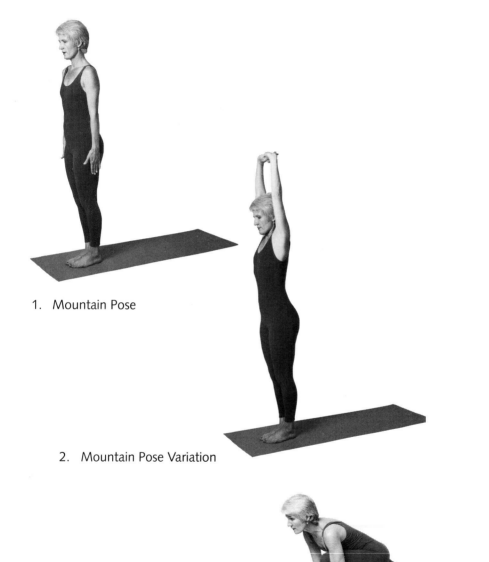

1. Mountain Pose

2. Mountain Pose Variation

3. Lunge, right leg back

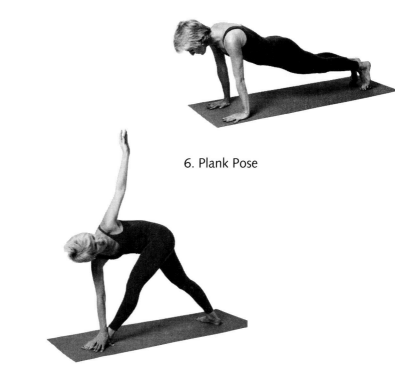

6. Plank Pose

5. Standing Spinal Twist, on left side

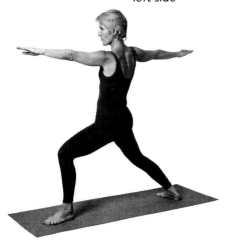

4. Proud Warrior

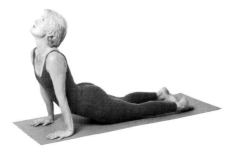

7. Up Dog

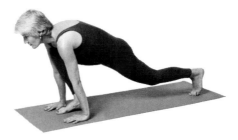

8. Lunge, left leg back

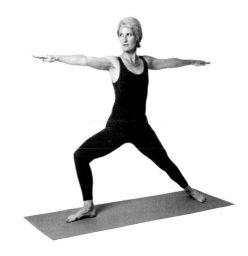

9. Proud Warrior

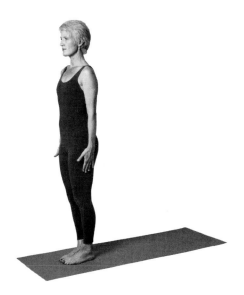

12. Mountain Pose

11. Standing Forward Bend

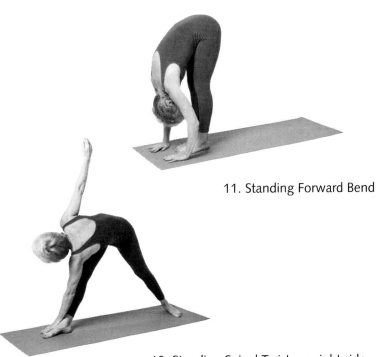

10. Standing Spinal Twist, on right side

SUN SALUTATION #4

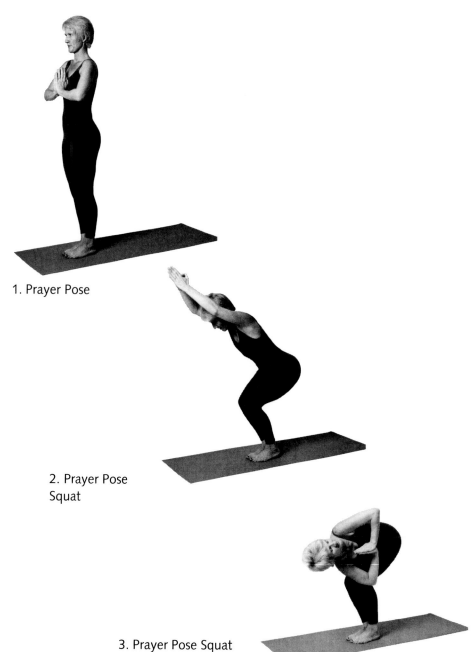

1. Prayer Pose

2. Prayer Pose Squat

3. Prayer Pose Squat Variation

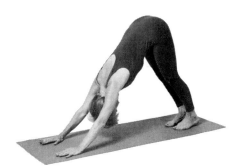

6. Down Dog

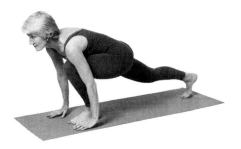

5. Lunge, right leg back

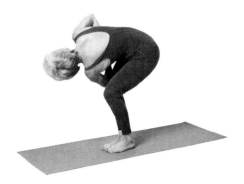

4. Both Sides

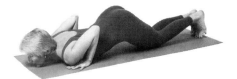

7. Plank Pose Variation (slowly lower your body)

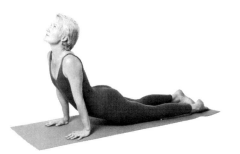

8. Up Dog

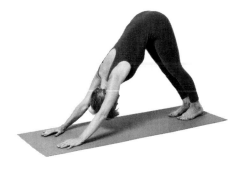

9. Down Dog

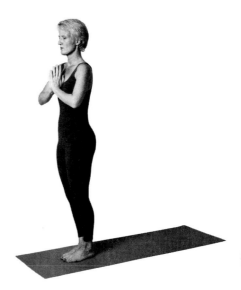

12. Prayer Pose

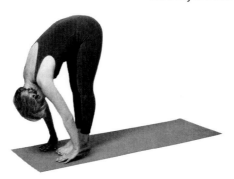

11. Standing Forward Bend

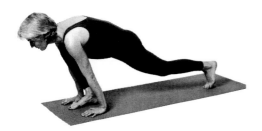

10. Lunge, left leg back

Sun Salutation #5

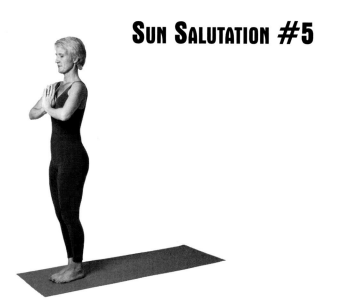

1. Prayer Pose

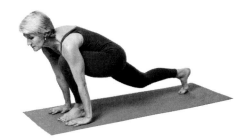

2. Lunge, right leg back

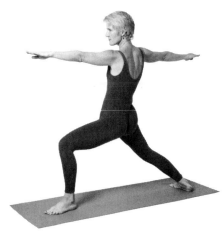

3. Proud Warrior

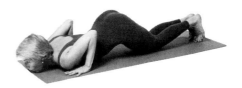

6. Plank Pose Variation

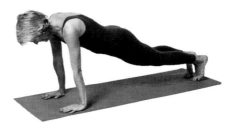

5. Plank Pose

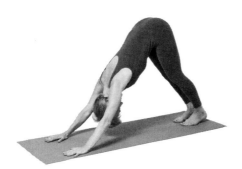

4. Down Dog

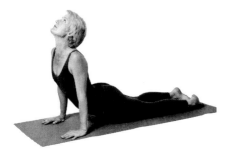

7. Up Dog

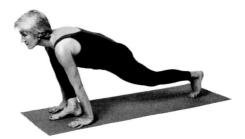

8. Lunge, left leg back

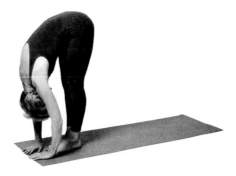

9. Standing Forward Bend

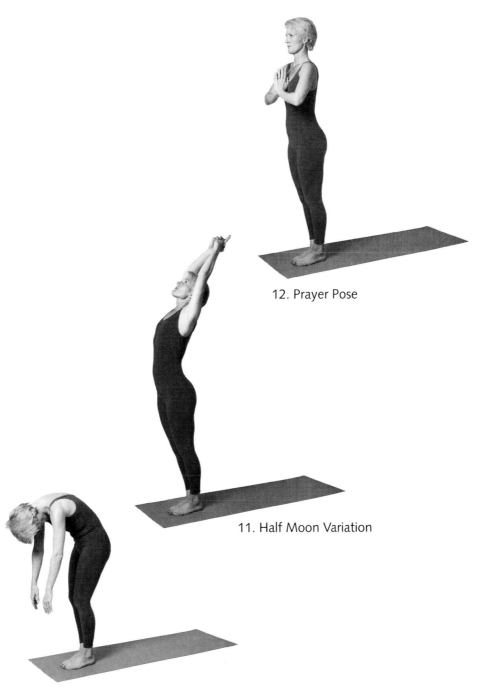

12. Prayer Pose

11. Half Moon Variation

10. Roll Up

SUN SALUTATION #6

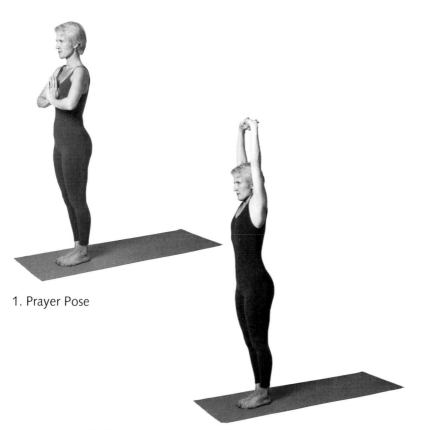

1. Prayer Pose

2. Mountain Pose Variation

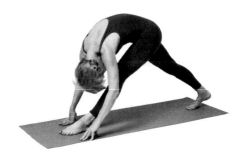

3. Runner's Lunge Variation, right leg back

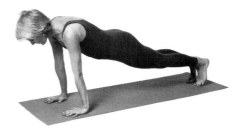

6. Plank Pose

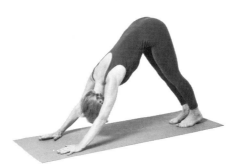

5. Down Dog

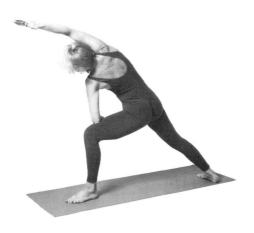

4. Warrior Side Stretch, right side

87

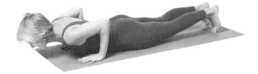

7. Reverse Push-up

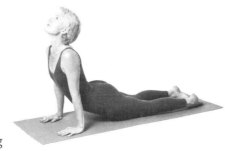

8. Up Dog

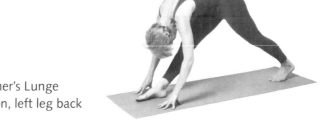

9. Runner's Lunge
Variation, left leg back

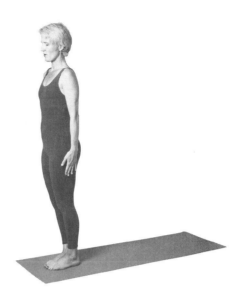

12. Mountain Pose

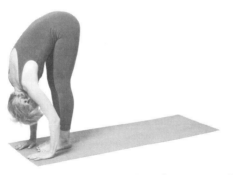

11. Standing Forward Bend

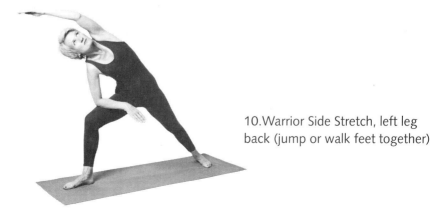

10.Warrior Side Stretch, left leg
back (jump or walk feet together)

89

SUN SALUTATION #7

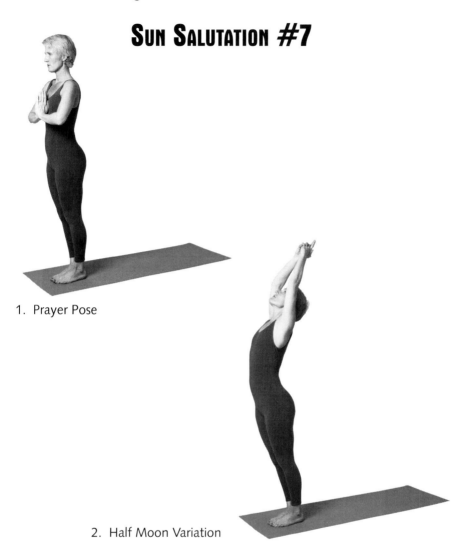

1. Prayer Pose

2. Half Moon Variation

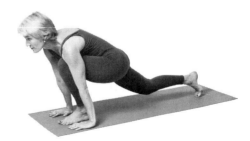

3. Lunge, right leg back

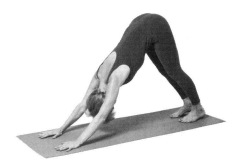

6. Down Dog

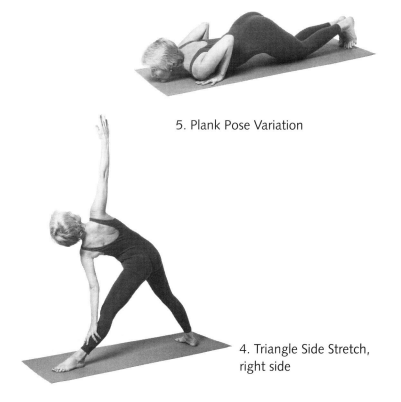

5. Plank Pose Variation

4. Triangle Side Stretch,
right side

91

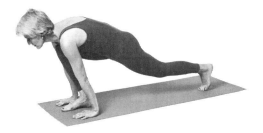

7. Lunge, left leg back

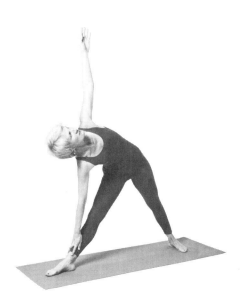

8. Triangle Side Stretch, left side (jump or walk feet together)

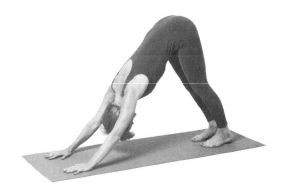

9. Down Dog

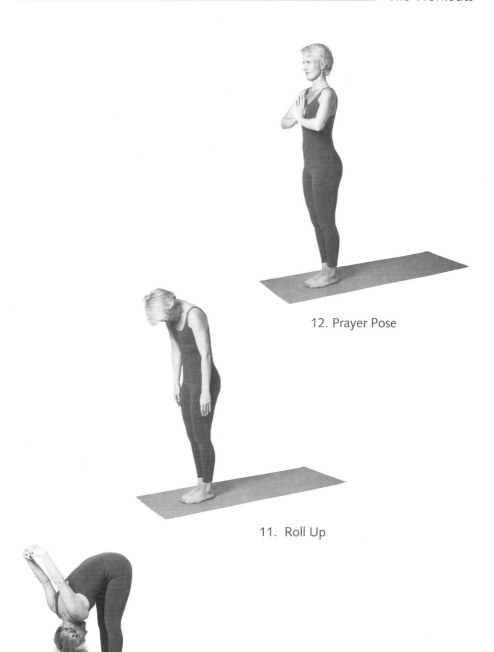

12. Prayer Pose

11. Roll Up

10. Standing Swimmer's Stretch

THE "I CAN'T BELIEVE IT'S YOGA" WORKOUTS

These are simplified workouts to do when you do not have time to perform a full class, which includes all the exercises in the book. Choose the workout that best suits your needs. You can vary these workouts as long as you warm up and save the more strenuous poses for the second half of the workout. Be sure to practice your Yoga routine three to four times a week, whether you do a 10-minute, 20-minute, or full hour program. Rotate workouts as needed to add variety to your fitness program.

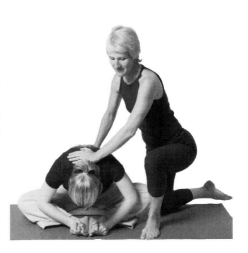

Once you become familiar with the poses, you can integrate additional Yoga exercises to the workouts. It is important to be sensitive to your own needs and limits. Breathing in and out through your nose encourages full breaths and helps warm your muscles.

10 Minute Workout

Sun Salutation #1
Sun Salutation #2
Sun Salutation #3
Seated Cross-Legged Position for three long breaths
Butterfly

10 Minute Workout

Sun Salutation #1
Sun Salutation #3
Sun Salutation #4

Mountain Pose
Rabbit
Cat Pose
Child's Pose
Hurdler Stretch, on both sides slowly
Seated Hamstring Stretch
Neck Rolls - 3x on each side

20 Minute Workout

Seated Cross-Legged Position
Fire Breath - 30x
Seated Stretch Forward
Seated Side Stretch - 3x
Inner Thigh Stretch
Standing Triangle Pose
Proud Warrior
Sun Salutation #3
Sun Salutation #5
Yoga Sit-ups - 10x
Pelvic Tilt
Plow
Shoulder Stand
Fish

Seated Workout

Seated Side Stretch
Seated Forward Stretch
Butterfly Position - Hold for three breaths
Hurdler Stretch - Repeat for a count of three to five breaths
     on each side
Inner Thigh Stretch - 3x
Boat Pose
Seated Spinal Twist
Cross-Legged Seated Position
Neck Rolls
Head Rolls
Fire Breath - 30x

10 Minute Morning Wake Up

Three Part Breath
Seated Forward Stretch
Cat Pose
Down Dog
Runners Lunge, both sides
Standing Forward Bend
Roll Up
Mountain Pose Variation
Triangle
Triangle Side Stretch, both sides
Proud Warrior, both sides

10 Minute Runner's Workout

(to do after running)
Dancer Pose
Standing Hamstring Stretch
Standing Swimmer's stretch
Roll Up
Warrior Pose
Warrior Side Stretch
Sun Salutation #5
Cross-Legged Seated Position
Modified Hurdler
Seated Forward Bend
Cat Pose - 5x
Pelvic Tilt
Yoga Sit-up
Cat Pose
Runner's Lunge
Standing Forward Bend
Roll Up
Mountain Pose

20 Minute Evening De-Stresser

Sun Salutation #5
Sun Salutation #7
Half Moon
Standing Hamstring Stretch
Triangle Side Stretch, both sides
Seated Cross-Legged Position
Seated Spinal Twist
Spinal Roll
Pelvic Tilt
Hip Socket Stretch
Hamstring Stretch
Cobra
Plow
Shoulder Stand
Fish Pose

5 Minute Office Revitalization Workout

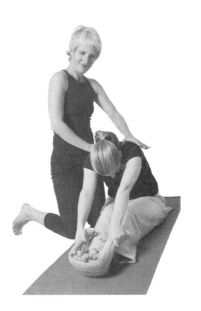

Half Moon
Half Moon Variation
Standing Forward Bend
Swimmer's Stretch
Roll Up
Seated Side Stretch, both sides
Seated Forward Stretch
Butterfly
Three Part Breath - 3x
Shoulder Rolls
Neck Rolls
Head Rolls

Part V: Relaxation

Now we finish the workout with a brief relaxation exercise.

I feel great. My muscles are so relaxed and my tension is gone.

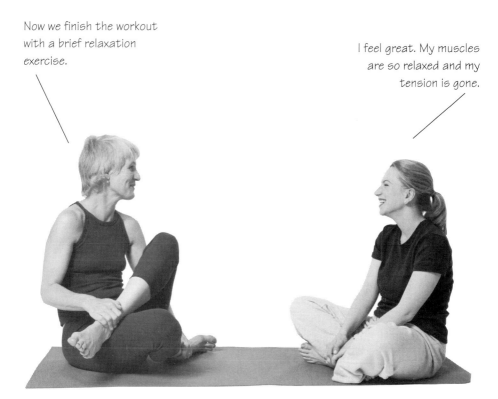

RELAXATION

Every practice of Hatha Yoga concludes with a relaxation pose. It can be as short as sitting cross-legged and focusing on your breath for a minute, to a 10 to 15 minute guided relaxation. Whichever you choose, be sure to sit in a room at a comfortable temperature, where you will not be disturbed. You can practice this guided relaxation after your Yoga workout, before you go to sleep, or even at the beach. You may find it helpful to have a friend record the following instructions for you to listen to on tape while you drift into a state of relaxation. This is the most efficient way to benefit from a guided relaxation.

Lie on the mat, close your eyes, or place an eye pillow over your eyes to block out light. *Try to focus inward.* Tell yourself there is no place you need to rush off to, and nothing to think about besides nourishing your body and mind for the next few minutes. Let yourself sink into a state of relaxation. Release the weight of your body into gravity. Feel your head, neck, and shoulders relax. Notice your elbows and hands let go into gravity. *Take the time to notice the benefits that you feel from your Yoga workout — the increase of circulation and awareness.*

Feel the muscles around your mouth relax, separate your back teeth, and release the jaw. Feel your breath naturally coming in through your nose and out through both your mouth and nose. Feel a widening across the chest as your breath fills your lungs. Release tiredness and tension as you exhale. Notice your back release into gravity, relaxing the muscles between your shoulder blades. *Feel yourself completely release all the tension in your body.* You are finished stretching and toning — now experience effortlessness. Give yourself time to focus inward and rejuvenate.

Feel your stomach lift as you inhale, and drop as you exhale. Feel the weight of your lower back and pelvis sink into gravity. Notice the increase of circulation in your hip sockets. Breathe as you sink into a deeper state of relaxation and inner awareness. Feel your right leg, knee, and ankle let go into gravity. Feel your left hip, knee, and ankle release. As you inhale, feel the circulation travel up the front of your body, across the face, and over the top of your head. As you exhale, feel the circulation travel down the back of your body to your feet. Repeat this inhale up the front and exhale down the back, as you release stress in all your muscles and tissues.

You will have more energy and be more centered from this relaxation. Roll to your side and sit up slowly, back into the Crossed-Legged Position. Notice your breathing. Take three long breaths as you inhale, hold, and exhale. Notice the light centered feeling that will stay with you throughout the day.

Ask yourself how you are feeling now, compared with how you felt at the beginning of the relaxation. Relaxation is a skill that has to be practiced and learned. By practicing it after your Yoga routine, you will be able to take these relaxation skills with you into everyday situations. You will find yourself taking a deep breath when you feel a stressful situation arising. These relaxation skills will also help your Yoga poses as you learn to focus from the inside out.

Practice these relaxation skills with your Yoga exercises or separately. *As with the Yoga poses, the more you practice, the more you will feel the benefits.*

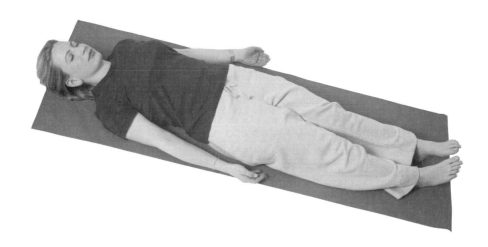

PART VI: NUTRITION

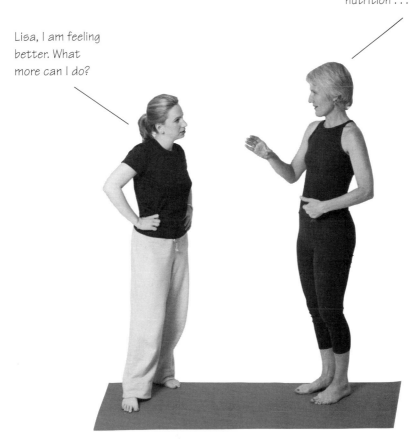

NUTRITION

Practicing Yoga regularly will increase your desire to eat a more nutritious and balanced diet. We practice Yoga to attain balance and energize ourselves, and we maintain a healthy diet for the same reasons. What we eat is reflected in our energy and muscle tone. By practicing Yoga, we get more in touch with how our mind and body feel. Eating nutritiously and doing Yoga prevent swings in energy and mood. The more you practice Yoga, the more you will crave healthier food. Much like Yoga, a healthy diet improves digestion and reduces stress.

The key to eating healthily is a balanced diet. Too much sugar can result in lower energy and reduced muscle tone. An all-protein or all-carbohydrate fad diet may work for a while, but creates imbalance in the long run.

Try to eat regular small meals, especially when exercising, with nutritious snacks in between. Stay away from excess meat, starches, processed foods, and sugar. Yoga will aid peristalsis and help cure some digestive disorders. A lowfat, mostly vegetarian diet is recommended. Try to eat more grains, vegetables, and fruits, keeping animal products to a minimum. Choose foods that offer the best balance of nutrients to meet your body's needs.

It is important to remember the concept of moderation when you are eating. Try to eat from all the main food groups each day. If one day you are traveling and eat fast food, you can equal it out at the next meal by eating a salad. Like Yoga, your diet should be about balance. If you eat a piece of cake, enjoy it and then drink an extra glass of water. Try not to be obsessive about whether you are eating correctly. Simply become more conscious of what you eat. Taking the time to eat slowly and enjoy the flavors will decrease the tendency to overeat.

Water

The most important element of your diet should be water. Drink at least eight glasses a day, and more if you are exercising regularly. Without food we can live for several weeks, without water we can only live for a few days. Water comprises more than one-half the body's weight. All cell processes and organ functions depend on water. Water is needed to keep food moving in our intestinal tract, eliminate wastes, prevent constipation, and regulate body temperature.

The body loses two to three quarts of water daily, more when exercising regularly, and this water needs to be replaced. We replenish some water through the food we eat. In warm weather, drink 16 to 20 ounces before your Yoga workout and eight ounces 15 to 20 minutes after the workout. Water keeps you hydrated and aids the metabolic functions balanced by the Yoga.

Explore New Foods

If you prefer eating in, read through cookbooks to find six new healthy and delicious recipes to add to your diet. If you are dining out, explore the healthy alternatives international restaurants have to offer, such as Italian pastas, Japanese soups and sushi, Chinese vegetables, Indian Curries, and Mexican vegetable tacos and burritos.

Average Intake

Based on guidelines established by The National Institutes of Health, you should balance the calories you consume with the calories you expend; the more active you are, the more calories you should take in.

It is recommended to have 20 to 30 grams of dietary fiber daily. Carbohydrates should make up 55% of your total caloric intake, low-fat protein sources should be 12% to 14%, and fat should account for 30% of your total calories, less than 10% of which should be saturated fats. Try to limit your dietary cholesterol intake to no more than 300 milligrams per day, and your salt intake to no more than one teaspoon.

Helpful Hints

- Stock your pantry with healthy snacks such as pretzels and trail mix for unexpected cravings.
- Steam, bake, or barbecue instead of frying.
- Use lowfat dressing.
- Eat fruit when you crave sugar.
- Reduce your consumption of coffee, tea, soda, and other caffenated beverages.

- Drink alcohol in moderation.
- Reduce your salt intake.
- Cut back on red meat, eating lowfat meats such as chicken and fish 2 to 3 times a week.
- Consider lowfat desserts.
- Put lemon on vegetables for flavor instead of butter.
- Do not shop for groceries on an empty stomach.
- Try to eat wholesome foods rather then compensating with supple ments.
- Instead of a milk shake, try a smoothy with yogurt, fruit, and ice as a tasty treat.
- Try to eat fruits and vegetables in season.
- Choose organic produce whenever possible.
- Eat whole grain rather than bleached flour products.

Average requirement:

Protein (Lean meat, poultry, fish, legumes, eggs, and nuts)	2 3 oz. servings
Calcium (Milk, yogurt, and cheese)	2 to 3 cups
Grains (Bread, cereal, rice, and pasta)	6 to 11 oz.
Fruits	3 to 4 servings
Vegetables (Leafy green vegetables) (Other vegetables)	1 cup 3 to 5 servings
Fats, oils, and sweets	eat sparingly

Nutrients

Food Source

Vitamins

Vitamin A ....dark green or yellow
vegetables, fruit, milk,
eggs

Vitamin B6 ....lean meats, poultry, fish,
whole grains, green
leafy vegetables, carrots,
potatoes

Vitamin B12 ....soy, lean meat, poultry

Vitamin C ....citrus fruits, papaya,
strawberries, melon

Vitamin D......................................soy products, dairy

Folicin ....green leafy vegetables,
orange juice, cantaloupes,
whole wheat

Vitamin E ....seeds, nuts, whole grains

Thiamin ....nuts, whole grains,
wheat germ

Riboflavin......................................milk, cheese, green leafy
vegetables

Niacin..fish, lean meats, peanuts,
whole grains

Minerals

Calcium ....dairy products, whole
grains, leafy vegetables

Phosphorus ....milk, cheese, lean meats

Iron ....oysters, spinach, beans

Iodine..sea vegetables

Magnesium ....nuts, seafood, whole
grains, dried beans, peas

A Final Note . . .

Begin practicing Yoga—the benefits that practicing Yoga has on your body and mind will carry over to many aspects of your life.

Start doing Yoga regularly—three or more times per week. You will see and feel many positive results.

Look through this book again and again. Take the time to read the explanations of the exercises. Choose to practice Yoga each week. Try to fit in a routine of Yoga at the gym, before you set out to work, or at the end of the day. You'll discover that the more you practice Yoga the better you'll feel.

With so many benefits, it is no wonder that once you start, you'll want to make Yoga an important part of your life.

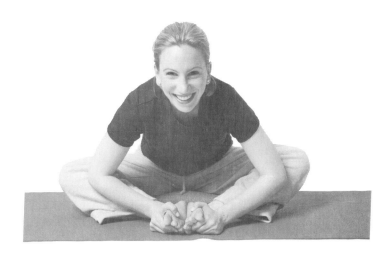

MEET THE AUTHOR

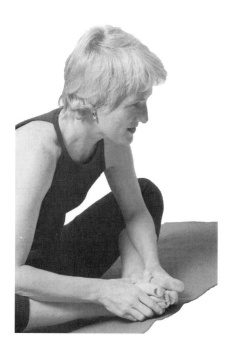

Lisa Trivell is a certified exercise and Yoga instructor, as well as a licensed massage therapist. For 15 years, She has taught Yoga in New York City and East Hampton in corporations, schools, and her private practice. She is certified by the International Fitness Professionals Association (IFPA) and the American Aerobics Associations International/ International Sports Medicine Association (AAAI / ISMA).

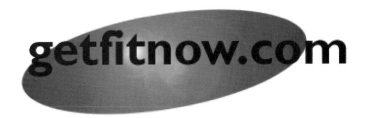

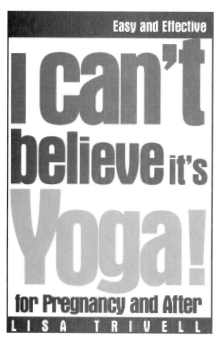

I Can't Believe It's Yoga for Pregnancy and After

I Can't Believe It's Yoga for Pregnancy shows women that yoga is the best way to stay in shape and prepare for childbirth. By relieving stress and discomfort, yoga is a safe, natural alternative for expectant mothers (and fathers too!). Beautifully photographed, with exercises for every stage of pregnancy. Also included are breathing exercises and relaxation techniques that can be used during labor and childbirth, plus specific postpartum exercises to help women restore their level of fitness and muscle tone.

Lisa Trivell has been a licensed massage and exercise therapist for over 18 years. She is a certified personal and yoga trainer by the International Fitness Professionals Association (IFPA). Lisa has been teaching yoga to pregnant women for the last three years.

ISBN 1-57826-046-9 $14.95

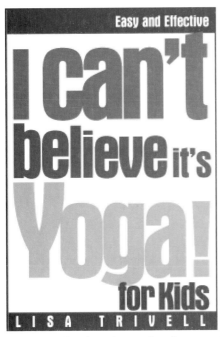

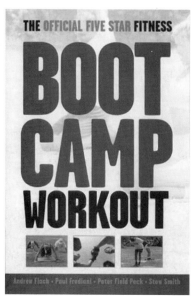

The Official Five Star Fitness Boot Camp Workout

Written by Andrew Flach, Paul Frediani, Stew Smith
Photographed by Peter Field Peck

The Official Five Star Fitness Boot Camp Workout presents a total body fitness program combining strength, endurance, flexibility, and cardio-conditioning. From coast to coast, everyone's discovering this "no frills," high energy approach to fitness.

The Official Five Star Fitness Boot Camp Workout will show you how to build a strong foundation for life-long fitness. Detailed, progressive 6-week workout plans for beginner, intermediate, and advanced workout warriors are featured. Minimal exercise equipment is required.

Whether you want to get strong, lose weight, increase your energy, or just have a fun workout, *The Official Five Star Fitness Boot Camp Workout* is the answer!

$14.95 ISBN: 1-57826-033-7

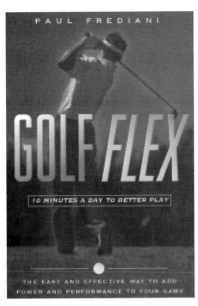

Crunch® Fitness Series

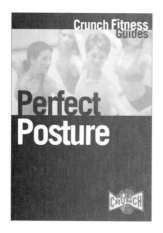

Throughout the country Crunch® is synonymous with the ultimate in fitness and exercise. From New York to LA, Crunch Fitness Centers have helped hundreds of thousands of Americans get in shape and stay in shape. With their unique lifestyle approach to fitness and their philosophy of "no judgments" on your lifestyle, Crunch is the choice of men and women, and who want to exercise their right to fitness.

Crunch is a major national chain of fitness centers. Their brand is widely recognized through a daily television exercise show on ESPN and through their videos and fitness apparel. Their upscale, user-friendly gyms are located in New York, Los Angeles, San Francisco, Miami, Chicago, and Tokyo.

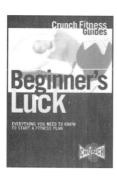
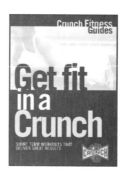
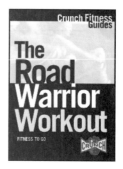

Also available in the Crunch Fitness Series

Perfect Posture

Good posture is very beneficial in a variety of ways–it can make you look better, feel better, and helps relieve a wide range of muscle and spine related complaints. The Crunch Perfect Posture book presents a combination of exercises, stretches and "Americanized" yoga techniques that will lead you to improved posture.

Also included are tips on selecting a mattress, the proper way to sit, how to prevent back injuries, and breathing exercises to help your spine and back.

$14.95 ISBN 1-57826-040-X

Workouts for Workaholics

Maintaining fitness on the job will help you work more productively, deal better with physical and emotional stress, and reduce sickness. This book shows you how to find the time at work to keep in shape. Includes exercises that can be done at your desk in business attire, relaxation techniques to fight stress, nutrition tips, and scheduling plans to get you out of the workplace and to a workout with the least amount of disruption.

$14.95 ISBN 1-57826-041-8

On Your Mark. Get Set. Go!
Training for your first marathon.

The marathon is the crown jewel of running. 26.2 miles of exhilaration and sometimes agony. This book is designed to get the novice, recreational runner from the starting line to the finish line. In keeping with Crunch's philosophy, there's no judgment on your finishing time, we just want you to finish. Covers everything to get you in shape mentally and physically including nutrition, detailed training schedules, exercises and stretches, the right equipment, dealing with pain and avoiding injuries.

$14.95 ISBN 1-57826-050-7

**Available in bookstores everywhere,
order toll free at 1-800-906-1234
or online at getfitnow.com.**

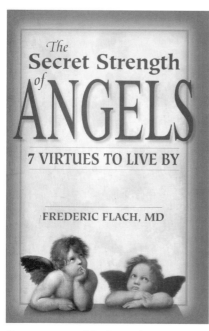